Foisted upon the Government?
State Responsibilities, Family Obligations,
and the Care of the Dependent Aged
in Late Nineteenth-Century Ontario

While government officials in the 1890s claimed that forcing families to take responsibility for caring for the aged was in the interest of the elderly, Edgar-André Montigny reveals that government policy had more to do with saving money than a desire to serve the aged. He provides a harsh critique of Ontario government policies toward the elderly and their families at the end of the nineteenth century and highlights similarities between what happened in the 1890s and current policy reforms in the area of long-term care.

Montigny argues that government played a central role in determining how society viewed the elderly and family obligations to them. Using census data, municipal records, and institutional case files, he demonstrates that the government created and promoted an image of the aged population that bore little resemblance to reality and manipulated the concept of family obligations to justify policies to reduce social-welfare costs. The effect of these policies, passed in the name of helping the elderly and their families, was almost universally negative.

By dispelling the myths that continue to influence public policy concerning the aged, Montigny provides a useful warning of the negative consequences of policies that are enacted to cut costs rather than to serve the population they are supposed to help.

EDGAR-ANDRÉ MONTIGNY is a post-doctoral fellow at Trent University.

McGILL-QUEEN'S/HANNAH INSTITUTE STUDIES IN THE HISTORY OF
MEDICINE, HEALTH, AND SOCIETY
Series Editor: S.O. Freedman and J.T.H. Connor

Volumes in this series have been supported by the Hannah Institute
for the History of Medicine.

Foisted upon the Government?

State Responsibilities,
Family Obligations,
and the Care of the
Dependent Aged
in Late Nineteenth-
Century Ontario

EDGAR-ANDRÉ
MONTIGNY

McGill-Queen's University Press
Montreal & Kingston · London · Buffalo

© McGill-Queen's University Press 1997
ISBN 0-7735-1616-6

Legal deposit fourth quarter 1997
Bibliothèque nationale du Québec

Printed in Canada on acid-free paper.

This book has been published with the help of a grant
from the Humanities and Social Sciences Federation of
Canada, using funds provided by the Social Sciences
and Humanities Research Council of Canada.

McGill-Queen's University Press acknowledges the
support received for its publishing program from
the Canada Council's Block Grants program.

Canadian Cataloguing in Publication Data

Montigny, Edgar-André
    Foisted upon the government?: state responsibilities,
    family obligations, and the care of the dependent aged
    in late nineteenth-century Ontario
    (McGill-Queen's/Hannah Institute studies in the
    history of medicine, health and society; 6)
    Includes bibliographical references and index.
    ISBN 0-7735-1616-6
    1. Aged – Government policy – Ontario – History –
    19th century. 2. Aged – Home care – Government
    policy – Ontario – History – 19th century. 3. Aged –
    Ontario – Social conditions. I. Title. II. Series.
    HV1475.06M66 1997   362.6'09713'09034
    C97-900352-0

This book was typeset by Typo Litho Composition
Inc. in 10/12 Sabon.

*In memory of Verna (Watters) Montigny
(1928–93)*

Contents

Figures and Tables

TABLES

Preface

I was not alone in preparing this book. Numerous individuals offered their time, expertise, advice, and, most of all, their support, encouragement, and patience.

The book began as a research paper for a doctoral seminar and was undertaken at the suggestion of Professor Chad Gaffield. At the time I was planning to write a thesis dealing with inheritance and migration patterns in nineteenth-century Quebec. My preliminary research had aroused a certain interest in the elderly, but it was not until I completed my paper for Professor Gaffield that I was motivated to change thesis topics and focus my attention upon the aged. The resulting thesis was completed at the University of Ottawa in 1994 and later was revised to become this book.

The faculty and staff of the University of Ottawa history department provided me with ample intellectual and emotional support during the preparation of my thesis. In particular, I am indebted to Donald Davis, Chad Gaffield, Lawrence Jennings, Michael Piva, and Francine Legace. Most of all, however, I must express my appreciation to my supervisor, Beatrice Craig. Her patience, practicality, and friendship helped me through the many crises doctoral candidates are prone to suffer.

I could not have completed my research without the assistance of the reference staff at the Archives of Ontario, in particular Karen Bergsteinsson, Leon Wormski, and Stormi Stewart. Just as important to me were my friends, both academics and non-academics, who, as a group, supported me in various ways. For the most part, they listened. They allowed me to babble on about my research, my discoveries, my theories, and my frustrations. Clare Dale stands out as one of the most constant and indispensable members of this group. As well, my partner Roger not only provided me with emotional support but developed a remarkable capacity for listening to me drone on about government policies, families, and the aged without allowing his eyes to glaze over.

I must also thank those people whose advice and suggestions helped produce the final version of the manuscript, namely Andrew Achenbaum, Donald Davis, James Struthers, David Thomson, and the three anonymous reviewers who prepared reports for the Social Sciences and Humanities Research Council of Canada (SSHRCC). Finally, this book would never have appeared without the support of the SSHRCC's Aid to Scholarly Publications Program and the cooperation and assistance of the team at McGill-Queen's University Press.

My greatest thanks, however, go to my parents. Anything I accomplish in life is largely due to the efforts of my mother and father. Their encouragement and love gave me the confidence to pursue my goals and their unending support, both emotional and financial, made it possible for me to succeed. No one was more fully behind me than my mother. At times she appeared more excited about my eventual graduation than I was. She often joked about being able to tell everyone about "my son the doctor." Her unexpected death only months before my thesis defence was a profound loss. It is to her that I dedicate this book. I only regret that she is not here to see it.

Foisted upon the Government?

Introduction

Western societies are entering a crucial period of debate about the future of the welfare state in which the rights and obligations of individuals, families, and communities must be reassessed. Much of the debate should, of necessity, focus on the entitlements of the aged and the distribution of resources between one generation and the next.[1] It is clear that the aged have already become a subject of concern. Many argue, however, that current discussions have barely touched upon the true complexity of the issues involved.[2]

According to newspapers, Statistics Canada, or any one of a number of publications about pensions, health care, or the economy, our society is currently faced with a major crisis: the crisis of an aging population. Politicians, economists, and journalists across North America and Europe have noticed that their societies are aging and they have responded with shock, treating the growth of the aged population as an unprecedented crisis of alarming proportions.[3] As Robert Evans explains, in countries like Canada, which are passing through a major demographic transition and shifting to a much older as well as slow growing or even static population, the individual experience of aging is easily projected as a "crisis."[4] This anxiety has been exacerbated by the dismal state of Western economies in recent years.

Population aging has become a major cause of concern not only in the realm of health care[5] but throughout all social-welfare fields. The most significant policy shift generated by the notion of impending "crisis" has been an overall re-evaluation of the level of responsibility that Western states wish to assume for the dependent portion of certain groups, particularly the elderly. In short, the combination of population aging and fiscal crisis has been used in various ways to justify the state's abdication of many of its responsibilities for the dependent aged and placing the burden of their support on the family and the local community.[6]

use of examples?

In the United States, for example, a variety of social and economic problems have been defined in terms of "the crisis of the aging population." It is frequently assumed that present-day economic difficulties are at least partly the result of growing numbers of aged people who, as "heavy consumers of welfare services," make unreasonable demands upon public funds.[7] The elderly, it is reported, are "busting the budget."[8] As a result, they have been described as a "major reason for the United States's economic problems."[9]

But they were the gross contributor.

Carroll Estes argues that the framing of the issue of an aging population in "crisis" terms has served two purposes. First, such rhetoric has justified the roll-back of state benefits for the aged. More significantly, however, the image of an impending crisis has stimulated a renewed interest in the idea of enforcing familial responsibility and insisting that family care be used as a substitute for state-provided services. For instance, under the administration of Ronald Reagan, the number of days a person was eligible for care under medicare was reduced. The immediate impact of this policy change was to shift more than 21 million days of care from the formal hospital-care system to the informal care of the home and the family.[10]

Similarly, the British government, in an attempt to reduce public expenditures in the field of public welfare, health, and social security, has, since the 1970s, increasingly emphasized the notion of "supporting the family" in an attempt to encourage families to assume a greater degree of responsibility for their members. This trend has been justified by gloomy predictions concerning the inevitable collapse of the country's caring services because of the aging of the population and the increased burden on state services which this is believed to represent.[11]

Why et than?

While these trends are not as dramatic in Canada, concern over population aging is evident. As early as 1979, the Institute for Research on Public Policy issued a report which spoke of population aging as "an increasingly difficult political problem and a continuing drain upon public resources."[12] As a result of such reports it is now commonly assumed that the old are "a burden to society."[13] Consequently, both concern over the impact of population aging and the need for fiscal restraint have resulted in an increasing emphasis on the idea of family care.[14] As in England and the United States, government policies aimed at providing care for the dependent aged are being based upon the assumption that, in the future, families will provide a greater degree of care for the elderly than is currently the case. While most of these policies are depicted as representing state support for the aged, in reality they are attempting to redefine the boundaries between family obligations and state responsibilities by placing a far greater share of the burden of care on the family.[15] In Ontario, recent reforms in long-term-

Who said they were a state responsibility in the first place

care policies appear to be following a similar course, reducing government spending on the aged and transferring responsibility for older generations from the state to younger generations.

Although policies that reduce government spending on the elderly are most often viewed as attacks upon them, it is clear that this is a one-sided view; the issue is far more complex. David Thomson argues that any analysis of social policies and government spending must take the generation factor into account. He points out that modern welfare states have not treated different generations equally and that, despite the current rhetoric concerning how poorly the aged are being treated by western states, today's elderly have been one of the most favoured generations ever, benefiting far more than any previous generation from government spending on social programs, tax reforms, and economic policies. What is more, they are likely much more fortunate in this regard than any future generation of elderly will be.[16]

Many age-specific benefits were instituted only in recent decades and, notwithstanding the protests of seniors' groups, current cutbacks have come nowhere near to erasing the massive gains the aged have made since the 1970s.[17] Thomson argues further that most of the increased spending on the aged has been financed by the generation born after 1950. In this sense the debate over services for the aged involves more than a discussion of the rights and entitlements of the aged; it also involves issues of generational equality. The changing relationship between the state and the elderly does not affect only the aged. In most cases, Thomson argues, later-born generations pay inordinately for the services governments offer the aged. The later-born, therefore, have every right to demand a reassessment of the current distribution of resources between generations.[18]

Clearly, more information concerning the relationship between the state, the aged, and the family is needed before current discussions can address the full range of complex issues involved in debates over the rights, entitlements, and obligations of individuals, families, communities, and generations. It is the purpose of this book to contribute some of that information by placing the changing relationship between the state, the family, and the aged in a historical context. The analysis examines government policy concerning the care of the dependent aged in late-nineteenth-century Ontario, focusing particularly upon policies relating to long-term care.

In the most basic sense, long-term care involves the care of those who, because of illness, infirmity, or mental or physical disability, are unable to provide for themselves all of the things they need to survive. Although persons of any age may require support, traditionally it has been the provision of services to the elderly that has dominated debates on long-term care. There are a variety of methods by which long-term care can be provided for people, but, until recently, institutional care has been the main focus of both public spending and legislation.

Information about the particular impact policy changes in this field have had on generational issues is not available. Government bureaucrats in the last century certainly did not mention issues of generational equality. For this reason, a specific study of how social policies in the past affected different generations is not possible. This study will, however, explore the state's use of the notion of family obligations in relation to the care of the dependent aged. Since that notion was often employed to transfer a greater degree of responsibility for the care of the aged onto younger generations, it should be understood to imply a certain redistribution of resources between age cohorts that has a more negative impact on one generation than on others. The analysis offered here reveals not only how the concept of family obligations has been perceived and used by the state in Ontario but also under what conditions the boundaries between state responsibilities and family obligations have shifted.

Such a study is important for several reasons. Although there have been several critiques of current long-term-care policies in both Ontario and Canada in general,[19] almost none of these studies include any meaningful historical perspectives. Yet an understanding of the historical precedents to today's debates can shed much light upon the various roles played by the state and the family in caring for the aged. Long-term-care or institutional-care policies are also issues that reflect both sides of the debate concerning the entitlements and obligations of the aged. On the one hand, reductions in state spending on caregiving for the dependent aged can be interpreted as an attack upon their rights and entitlements. Conversely, since reductions in government spending in the field of institutional or long-term care for the aged often involve placing a greater share of responsibility upon families and later-born generations, such actions can be seen as examples of how state social policy has distributed rewards and obligations unevenly between generations. This study will suggest, however, that in many cases reductions in government spending on caregiving for the dependent aged negatively affect all generations concerned without offering any clear benefits to the state.

An examination of current debates from a historical perspective is also necessary to develop public policies that are based on facts and realities instead of myths and assumptions. Several myths dominate discussions about the elderly and their families and the relationship between various generations and the state.[20] Three in particular are relevant to any discussion of the evolution of public policies affecting the aged. The first is that the bulk of the aged population is ill, infirm, destitute, and dependent. Secondly, it is frequently asserted that current debates about the care of the aged are unprecedented simply because in the past there were too few aged people for their care to become a public concern. Finally, it is widely accepted that public support for the aged originally became necessary because sometime late in the last century families began to refuse to provide sufficient amounts of care and support to their aged kin. Only a detailed historical analysis of concerns about the aging of the population and the policy debates regarding the degree of responsibility the state should assume for the dependent aged can help to dispel these myths and permit legislators to develop policies that are based upon the true circumstances of the aged and their families.

Moreover, only a historical perspective can reveal the degree to which public policy itself helped create these myths. Such a study can also detail how both family obligations and old-age dependency have been socially constructed and determined by state-policy decisions. Neither the degree of care society expects families to provide for the aged nor the degree of need experienced by the aged population has been constant.[21] Both have been affected by a variety of social forces. Through social-policy decisions, however, the state can exert a profound influence over decisions concerning what type of care is provided for the aged and who should provide it.[22] The government, therefore, plays a central role in determining how individuals and society have viewed the dependent aged and the family's obligations towards them.

Exactly what this role has been has been determined by three factors: beliefs about the level of need and dependency among the aged population, the degree of concern about the size of that population, and the level of the state's anxiety about fiscal restraint. In periods when the state fears a massive increase in the size of the aged population and the assumption is that this population will be highly needy and dependent, it is likely that the state will attempt to reduce its responsibilities for this group. If these fears coincide with a period of fiscal restraint, it is almost certain that the state will abdicate a large portion of its responsibilities in this area and elect to emphasize family obligations in order to justify transferring these responsibilities to the family. A study of Ontario in the 1890s will highlight this process and offer some insights into current debates over the reform of long-term-care policies.

It has been proven that a knowledge of the historical precedents relating to present-day policy debates on care for the aged can help legislators appreciate that the options facing society today are similar to those considered, tried, and often discarded by previous generations which also had to grapple with the same problems.[23] More important, researchers in England have demonstrated that social policies initiated in the nineteenth century have had an enduring impact on the content and implementation of public programs. For this reason, Jill Quadagno explains that "it is only by understanding the legacies of social policy we have inherited that we can begin to make sense of present policy debates. In order to formulate policy change for the future we must re-evaluate the validity of assumptions imbedded in programmes that are a legacy from the past."[24] This is especially true of programs directed towards the aged. Authors such as Allan Walker and Peter Townsend contend that the dependency of the aged today is not a natural occurrence due to the intrinsic characteristics of old age but a consequence of social policies, many of them first initiated during the final decades of the nineteenth century, which have created and reinforced the dependency of aged people.[25] As Townsend argues: "Society creates the framework of institutions and rules within which the general problems of the elderly emerge and are indeed, manufactured. Decisions are being taken every day, in the management of the economy and in the maintenance and development of social institutions which govern the position which the elderly occupy in national life."[26] Similarly, John Myles asserts that the social and economic circumstances of Canada's aged are determined by "public policy, rather than market forces."[27] Not only has public policy had a major impact on the income of the aged but it has also played a significant role in determining who the aged have turned to for support when they found that their incomes were inadequate to provide the care and support they needed to survive. It is clear, therefore, that it is public policy and not any innate sense of family obligations which regulates the kinds and amounts of assistance the aged can expect to receive from their families and what types of support they are likely to receive eventually from the state.

FAMILY OBLIGATIONS AND THE STATE

Family obligations and government policy have long been closely related. In terms of the degree to which family obligations are valued or enforced, as well as the nature and extent of what families are obligated to do and for whom, government policy has frequently played a major role in determining what society believes is normal, practical, and acceptable. As Janet Finch explains: "In a society where there are a range of different and sometimes conflicting norms and values about family life, social policies represent a very public statement of a particular position which can potentially be backed up by sanctions and it is likely that they occupy a distinctive role in shaping what is often referred to as the climate of opinion."[28] This is an important point given that governments, especially in social-welfare states, have a vested interest in defining what structures of support should exist in families and how people should think about their family responsibilities.[29] Most social policy in western states has focused upon the individual rather than the family. The dominant belief has been that individual citizens have a right to adequate resources for survival and that the claims which they make to secure these are upon the community as a whole rather than upon their own families.[30] The state acts as a mechanism by which such claims are made by collecting taxes and redistributing resources. It is within the state's power, however, to modify the circumstances under which resources are redistributed in such a way as to ensure that people rely on their families rather than the state to ensure their survival.[31] The state can also alter policies in a fashion that favours one generation and penalizes another.[32] When it comes to the care of the dependent aged, the concept of family obligations is often the tool used by the state to enact such policy changes.

This has been evident in Canadian social policy. Susan Watt argues that the state's interpretation of the family's responsibilities towards the aged have varied over time depending upon the condition of the state's treasury. She explains that, in the construction of social policy, various models of family have been used. Each model carries with it certain assumptions about the role of the family in the care of its dependent members and the degree to which the state should assist families in their caring functions. When economic times are good, models that accept a large degree of state responsibility for the aged have been employed; in bad economic circumstances, models that impose a much greater burden on the family have been initiated.[33]

Thus, as governments attempt to reduce their social-welfare expenditures during periods of fiscal restraint, the aged increasingly are spoken of as a "social problem" and it is decided that families must do more if the state is to advert a "crisis." Over time these concerns evolve into debates over how the state can force families to assume their proper degree of responsibility for their aged kin. In combination, the images of "social problem," "crisis," and family obligation become the justification for the implementation of policies which, to varying degrees, reduce social spending on services for the aged, restrict access to services for those aged people who have kin, and enforce various types of familial responsibility for the aged. It is within the framework of justifying such policies that myths about the aged emerge: the notion of old-age dependency, the claim that there was no aged population in the past, and the idea that families somehow have ceased to carry their fair share of responsibility for the aged.

THE AGED AS A SOCIAL PROBLEM

The image of the aged as a "social problem" usually appears during periods of genuine or at least perceived population aging; indeed, population aging and panic over an impending social crisis often go hand in hand. Yet the number of older people in a population does not necessarily have to be increasing for population aging to be perceived as a potential threat. This claim is supported by the findings of Brian Gratton, who studied the aged in the United States, and Jill Quadagno, who examined public policies towards the elderly in England. Both discovered that intense public concern over growth in the size of the aged population arose independently of any significant alterations in the demographic status of the elderly.[34] It is clear, then, that the concept of the aged as a social problem is based more on people's attitudes, perceptions, and assumptions than on actual facts.[35] This is because, as Sheila McIntyre points out, a social problem consists of two components, an objective condition and a subjective definition. Once an issue is perceived to be a problem by the public, policy makers, or administrators, the objective condition is often of secondary importance.[36]

The subjective construction of population aging becomes apparent when one notes that even when populations have been truly aging the increase in the numbers of old people in and of itself has not often been a cause for concern. The aged are not viewed as a "social problem" until it is also believed that most old people are destitute and dependent upon other people for their survival. Population aging, therefore, is not the problem. It is the increasing burden on the public purse that they are believed to represent that creates the "social problem" and the panic over an impending "crisis." Even this potential burden is not in itself necessarily sufficient cause for panic. It is mainly during periods of fiscal restraint that the image of an increasing outlay of funds for a growing population of dependent old people causes policy officials to depict population aging or the aged themselves as a "social problem."[37]

THE CRISIS OF AN AGING POPULATION

Susan McDaniel argues that it is not by accident that demographic aging has emerged as an important guiding paradigm in recent Canadian public-policy discussions and research or that the aged have become a popular subject in magazines, newspapers, and television and radio talk shows. Rather, the invocation of the population-aging paradigm, she argues, "enables politicians, business leaders, employers and the public to search for answers to the riddle of social problems in the realm of population structure."[38] This trend also allows policy makers *) perhaps* to blame social problems on population aging rather than searching for more viable explanations. More important, the problem of our aging population has taken on greater significance as various government officials and public agencies have responded to the economic crisis which has dominated public-policy debates in recent years. Herbert Northcott explains that this "crisis" definition of population aging arises because it serves the interests of certain groups in society.[39] By creating or at least fueling the fear that has come to characterize much of the public-policy debate surrounding the provision of services for the elderly, governments can help generate public support for policies that involve reducing public spending on the aged.

Y ✳ Government has at least partially funded current literature which helps support the image of the aged as a social problem.[40] Entire fields of study, such as social gerontology, have emerged as national concerns about the social and economic consequences of population aging have prompted increased spending on social-science research concerned with the elderly.[41] Much of this research has focused upon the potential problems associated with what many people feel will be an increase in the proportion of non-productive and dependent persons in their midst.[42] Recently, Statistics Canada reported that the population is growing older faster than predicted and that this may have "major social and economic implications." In particular, the report threatens that population aging will add to the "financial pressures of supporting the elderly, possibly requiring a shift in resources to that age group from the young."[43]

Despite significant evidence attesting to the high levels of social and economic independence among the aged, much of the current literature on aging emphasizes the dependency of the elderly upon the state, highlighting their needs as recipients of various forms of welfare and social assistance.[44] Northcott argues that this may be because, regardless of whether the conclusions have any relevance to those persons who are the object of discussion, the definition of the "problem," namely population aging, and the proposed solutions serve the vested interests of the problem-definers and the policy makers.[45] Similarly, journalist Thomas Walkom suggests that vote-seeking politicians are guilty of enacting cost-cutting policies which target the elderly in response to "simmering public resentment," rather than because the facts reveal that such actions are necessary.[46]

The frequent equation of growing numbers of aged people with growing numbers of dependent people creates a sense of panic concerning population aging and permits commentators to depict every increase in the size of the aged population as an automatic cause for alarm because it is assumed that such growth will bring with it enormous penalties in terms of human suffering and financial costs.[47] This is what Northcott describes as population-aging rhetoric, the primary goal of which is to persuade and convince people rather than inform them.[48] Only rarely does the rhetoric present objective information about current circumstances and historical trends.[49] Instead, the simple, but mistaken, translation of demographic projections into social realities is used to encourage the belief that the problem of social dependency exists just because the numbers in a particular age group are increasing.[50]

The truth is that the provision of services to the aged is not the problem. The real social problem is that Western economies are in a state of recession. Nevertheless, even if arguments about the crisis of an aging population are not correct or based on empirical analysis, it is easy to convince the public that the aged are dependent upon the state and that they represent an unreasonable burden upon the public purse. What becomes more important than scientific validity or determination of causality, Susan McDaniel asserts, is the setting in place of population aging as the unifying explanatory framework for previously inexplicable or unlinked problems.[51] More important, this type of argument is used to justify public policies which reduce services to the aged in the name of fiscal restraint and austerity.

While many emphasize that the aged are vulnerable in times of fiscal difficulties because they tend to be the largest single group in receipt of government assistance,[52] what is not so often mentioned is the degree to which the families of the aged are vulnerable and how often reductions in government spending in this area tend to involve sacrificing the interests of younger generations as much as those of the aged themselves. Government cutbacks in support for the aged often target those services that potentially can be provided by family members. Families, therefore, end up bearing the brunt of the state initiatives which reduce the amount of money spent on the aged. In this sense, the entire discussion about population aging, old-age dependency, and fiscal restraint can be interpreted as a debate over whether the family or the state should have primary responsibility for the care of the dependent aged.[53]

The problem with this debate is that it is guided by the image of the aged as a social problem which may bear little relation to the actual condition of the aged themselves. The debate is also clouded by the current emphasis on defending the rights of the aged without giving equal consideration to the rights and entitlements of the later-born, an approach that ignores the possibility of a conflict of interest between generations.[54] Hence, policies that are developed in this manner, especially those that redefine the relationship between the family and the state in the care of the aged, may not be based upon the real circumstances of either the aged or the later-born. Consequently, they may do little to meet the genuine needs of the aged, their families, or the state.

One does not have to search for long to discover that many of the assumptions upon which the image of the aged as a social problem is based are inaccurate and that much of the information which is used to justify the transfer of state responsibilities for the aged onto the family is also incorrect. For instance, despite the assumption that there were too few aged people in the past for them to become a concern of public officials, European societies have had to deal with population aging and the welfare costs associated with it from as early as the seventeenth century. While the recent growth of the aged population seems "unprecedented" in relation to the nineteenth century, and government publications have described it as a "new historical phenomenon,"[55] investigations of early periods indicate that the situation is not new. In England, at least, it was the unusually high fertility rates of the nineteenth century and the resulting youthful age structure which were unique and unprecedented. It appears that the twentieth century's population aging, rather than being abnormal, is merely a means by which the population can return to the demographic composition that was prevalent in earlier centuries.[56]

In the area of health care, reports of population aging creating a crisis in which "silver threads threaten to strangle the system"[57] seem to assume that the bulk of the aged population and certainly all people over the age of eighty-five require prolonged, intense, and expensive services from the health-care system. Based on this assumption, it is asserted that any growth in the numbers of old people will result in a corresponding increase in costs. Yet the fact is that, while there is a clear association between old age and disability, the vast majority of aged people are able to care for themselves either entirely without help or with only minimal support.[58] Even among the very old (those over the age of eighty-five), a recent study discovered that only one-third of the population required more than minimal assistance.[59] It has also been suggested that in the future the old may not require such varied or prolonged health care as many do today.[60] Most significantly, it has been demonstrated that the rising health-care costs so frequently blamed upon the growth of the aged population are largely due to a variety of trends within the medical industry which are rarely related to demographic change or any increase in the number of infirm old people. The availability of new technology, the manner in which services are delivered, and a tendency to over-medicate and over-hospitalize the aged, as well as dramatic price increases in the pharmaceutical and medical industry, have all contributed to rising health-care costs and are factors that are largely independent of population aging.[61]

Not only is much of the information currently being circulated about the aged inaccurate, but its ultimate impact has been to reinforce images and perceptions of the aged as a social problem rather than to promote a realistic understanding of their needs and circumstances. Such rhetoric can have significant ramifications for both the aged and their families, given the role images of panic and crisis can play in public-policy debates regarding the state's commitment towards caring for the dependent elderly. It is apparent, therefore, that a detailed analysis of the origins of our current images of the aged and the government policies that affect them is necessary.

In order to investigate the state's role in determining what obligations family members have had towards the aged and under what conditions these obligations have been redefined, the following chapters will examine the issue of the provision of care for the dependent aged in a historical context. First, the statements, assumptions, and perceptions of Ontario's nineteenth-century bureaucrats and legislators concerning the aged and their families will be presented and discussed. Then, the validity of these statements will be tested by comparing them to the actual condition of the elderly population in the 1890s. Finally, the historical information will be employed to offer suggestions as to the possible impact of current long-term-care reform upon the aged and their families. It is hoped that this overview of public policies affecting the aged and their families will provide an understanding of the role played by social policy in defining, not only the balance between the responsibilities of the state and the obligations of the family, but also the nature of the relationships between generations.

It was decided to study this issue on a provincial rather than a national level because welfare, poor relief, and institutional care – the main public-policy issues relating to the maintenance of the aged population – were, by the British North America Act of 1867, deemed to fall within provincial jurisdiction. For this reason, debates concerning the support and maintenance of the aged occurred at the provincial rather than the federal level. This point has been obscured by twentieth-century concerns over pensions and the development of pension legislation, which have caused most attention to be focused on federal policies. James Struthers, however, has pointed out that when a history of the aged in Canada is written, the bulk of the story will be local and provincial.[62]

Ontario has been chosen as the focus of this study for several reasons. An obvious one is that the province is currently in the midst of planning a major reorganization of health, social, and caregiving services for the aged and the disabled. As well, the Ontario government's

Strategies for Change has provided the most comprehensive articulation of where government thinking on the issue of long-term care in Canada is headed.[63] In the historical context, it was nineteenth-century Ontario where the issue of the aged as a social problem first appeared as a major concern of Canadian public officials and policy makers. During this period, Ontario was Canada's most populated and most industrialized province. It also boasted, as it does today, the nation's most developed government-supervised system of public welfare. Moreover, a comparatively rich variety of provincial and municipal sources allows one to explore the lives, needs, and conditions of the aged population at a local and personal level and to compare this information with that presented in government reports.

Unfortunately, no complete verbatim debates of the Ontario legislature have survived for the period under study. Only *Newspaper Hansard* reports on the activities of the legislature remain and these rarely mention issues related to the care of the dependent aged. Hence, one cannot determine how particular politicians felt about these issues or how party policies differed. There does exist, however, a wealth of information in the reports of various government officials, such as the inspector of prisons and public charities. For this reason, the government views presented here are actually the views of government bureaucrats rather than of individual politicians. Yet it is clear that government policy was based upon the recommendations of these officials. As the future premier George Ross stated in 1890, it was never the custom to present the reports to the house in detail; the recommendations of the bureaucrats concerning the funding and often the regulation of various charities and institutions were, for the most part, merely accepted and acted upon.[64] Such reports, then, offer a fairly accurate source for studying government social policy in the 1890s, particularly since the aged, a group rarely mentioned in the published accounts of the legislative debates, received a great deal of attention from various bureaucrats.

Despite the relative wealth of sources, there is a distinct lack of historical research concerning the condition of the aged or their families in Ontario or in the rest of Canada. For the purposes of this study, therefore, I have drawn extensively on the scholarship of England and the United States. These countries were chosen partly because they have produced the bulk of the literature on aging, family obligations, and social policy in the nineteenth century[65] and partly because, as Ann Shola Orloff has argued in her study of the development of pensions in Britain, Canada, and the United States, these three nations share "substantial similarities" which are commonly invoked in discussions of social-welfare policy. In particular, they share a common liberal culture and ideological heritage and democratic political systems.[66]

defending sources

TRUE BUT...

More specifically, much of nineteenth-century Ontario's political organization and social policy was based upon British models. The majority of the men who created and implemented public policy in the province were of British origin and often they supported and encouraged the preservation of British traditions and values. Ontarian society and political culture was not, however, a re-creation of that of Great Britain. The proximity of the province to the United States and the economic, social, and political links that developed between the two nations as a result also helped influence and mould the provincial identity. As Tamera Hareven points out, the American influences on Canadian social policy were important. "During the formative stages in Canadian welfare," she reports, "there was a consistent reliance on American experience."[67] As a result, Gordon Stewart explains, Ontario's political culture and public policies were based upon both British and American principles and philosophies.[68]

Another reason why a study of historical precedents for current policy initiatives in Ontario must use British and American studies as a reference is that in many cases those countries possess more complete and detailed records than those available for Ontario. On occasion, the existing records for Ontario do not permit a researcher to draw any firm conclusions. *Neg?* One can often do no more than point out that the records in Ontario suggest that the situation was either similar or contrary to that discovered by researchers in England or the United States who were able to draw more specific conclusion based on more complete records.

It is clear, then, that much can be learned by comparing and contrasting Ontario's public policies towards the aged with the approaches taken in both England and the United States. Yet one cannot assume that, because British or American policies influenced Ontario's legislators, social policies in Ontario always followed exactly the course taken by either of these two nations. While the trends and developments in Britain and the United States may be used as a guide for a study of Ontario's public policy towards the aged, it must be recognized that Ontario's approach to social issues had distinctive features.[69]

Balance

There are certain methodological problems associated with studying the history of policies and perceptions concerning the aged and the role of the family in their care. The first is determining exactly who qualifies as aged. There has always been a wide variety of ages, ranging between forty-five and seventy, at which people were deemed to be old.[70] In the past, the most commonly accepted point at which people were considered old was the age of sixty. John Demos found that in New England this was the age at which exemption from civic obligations took effect and ministers regularly described as old those members of their congregation who were over that age.[71] Similarly, as early as 1789, sixty was the age at which residents of Ontario were exempt from militia duty. Currently, however, sixty-five is the official age of retirement and therefore the age at which old age is considered to begin.

In light of these differences, it is difficult to compare the size and composition of nineteenth-century aged populations with those of today. As far as family obligations and home care are concerned, however, the differences are not as significant as they might appear on first glance. It is commonly accepted that sixty-year-olds today are far more active, healthy, and energetic than their counterparts from the 1890s. Since old-age disability tended to occur at an earlier age a century ago than it does now, in terms of the population who required support and care from their families, it may actually not be that problematic to compare the nineteenth-century over-sixty population with the current over-sixty-five population.

Even when one decides what age groups are elderly, it is sometimes difficult to determine who is included in these groups. Current records make it clear who is over the age of sixty-five. Historical records, however, are more ambiguous. To begin with, David Radcliffe points out that few people identified themselves as elderly by reference to their chronological age. Many, in fact, simply did not know their exact age.[72] For instance, George Emery notes that four hundred and twenty-one centenarians were listed in the 1871 census of Canada. The ages of only eighty-two of these people could be verified and, of these, only nine were actually over one hundred years old.[73]

These discrepancies between a nineteenth-century person's actual age and his or her reported age is easy to understand when one realizes that until recently there was little incentive for people to remember their exact age. It was only with the introduction of education and other age-based public services and benefits that both the recording of age and a person's awareness of that age became significant.[74] A 1908 *Punch* cartoon illustrates this point well. An aged woman is asked the date of her birth by a pension official. The woman replies, "Sure, there was no such thing as dates when I was born."[75]

In the nineteenth century, people described themselves or were described by others as old when they felt old or when their infirmities or frailty made it impossible for them to remain active. Hence, a large number of people who felt older than they were simply exaggerated their age. This tendency most certainly was emphasized as a person's health deteriorated.[76] It also appears that there was a class bias which determined how a person was referred to by others. The wealthy, although they may have been "advanced in years," were rarely described as old. "Old," it appears, was a term reserved for the poor. This also could have reflected the fact that the term "old" was related more to one's health than to one's age; the wealthy were inclined to remain healthy longer than manual labourers, who tended to become infirm at an earlier age.[77]

Considering that the term "old" was based on qualitative more than quantitative criteria, and that records which could confirm a person's age are not always available, it is often difficult to determine an individual's precise age. It is reasonable to assume, however, that anyone who perceived himself or herself to be old, or anyone who was perceived by others as old, was treated as such by their communities, regardless of their exact chronological age. In this sense, the treatment of people who were described by their contemporaries as being part of the aged population offers a valid indication of how old people were cared for or dealt with. For this reason, while anyone over the age of sixty shall be considered aged for the purposes of this study, those people who described themselves as old, or who were described as old by others, will be included as well even if quantitative records indicate that they were not actually over the age of sixty.

Once it is determined who is to be studied, one must decide what sources can be used to study them. Again, whereas literature on the current period is vast, easily accessible records dealing with the nineteenth century are not. This fact has had serious consequences not only for historical research but also for current public-policy decisions. Most of the easily accessible sources of historical information about the aged is contained in government-generated studies and reports relating to those aged people who required financial assistance, medical care, or institutional accommodation. These sources have led historians to focus their investigations on the destitute, infirm, and decrepit minority of the elderly population who were the recipients of public assistance and therefore the subjects of most nineteenth-century government policies and programs.

By relying on such information, historians have, perhaps unintentionally, conveyed the impression that this unfortunate group was representative of the entire aged population of the period. That was not so. Yet, though these people were exceptional in their poverty, dependence, and infirmity, they dominate almost all studies of the elderly in nineteenth-century Ontario. This has meant that the bulk of the information available to policy makers concerning the historical condition of the aged in Ontario has been data generated by other government officials, people who often had very specific political agendas. Such information has helped to reinforce the perception of the aged as a largely destitute, ill, and dependent group. Few have questioned either the validity of the data contained in these government reports on the aged or the motives of the officials and policy makers who produced them.[78] Rarely, for example, has anyone attempted to compare the actual condition of the aged population with the information found in government documents. Instead, most historians have accepted the statements of nineteenth-century officials at face value and so have perpetuated and reinforced the perceptions of these individuals and the assumptions about the aged population upon which most of their comments and policies were based. As well, few studies have attempted to investigate the degree to which the government had a vested interest in promoting the image of the aged as a predominantly destitute, ill, and dependent population. Nor do many Canadian authors explore how the government's construction of the aged as a social problem related to policy concerns about the level of responsibility the state wished to assume for this population.

Sources do exist which, although not directly or obviously related to the aged, contain information that permits an investigation of these issues. Despite assertions that old people were usually infirm and mentally incapacitated, diaries, letters, and biographies reveal that aged individuals frequently led active, productive lives. Census reports indicate that, contrary to government statements concerning the rising number of aged people who required public assistance, the portion of the elderly population inside institutions or receiving public aid grew little. Information about income levels for aged people reveal that, while the social workers and government officials decried the increasing incidence of poverty among the elderly, the bulk of the aged population had sufficient savings, property, and income to provide themselves with an adequate living. More important, all these sources provide testimony to the fact that, contrary to government pronouncements concerning the tendency of families to refuse to care for their aged kin, relatives provided a substantial degree of care for the elderly.

Even traditional sources, usually used to support government claims, can be employed in new ways to reveal that many statements made by institutional authorities and social commentators were inaccurate. Petitions for poor relief, often used as proof that the aged were destitute and dependent upon public relief, also provide evidence of the elderly's self-sufficiency and the degree to which the aged were cared for by family members, friends, and neighbours alike. Institutional records, normally cited as evidence that families were abandoning the aged in houses of industry and mental institutions, contain a wealth of information to the contrary. These records demonstrate that families cared for the aged as long as they were able and resorted to institutionalization only when all other options had been exhausted. They also show that what officials regularly regarded as acts of irresponsibility on the part of families were actually decisions forced upon them by the government policies, rules, and regulations which left them no alternative.

What emerges from a study of these records, finally, is a situation that was in many ways similar to that of the present. The government of late-nineteenth-century Ontario faced an economic crisis. Believing that the crisis was largely due to the costs of providing overly generous social benefits to the population, it concluded that spending in this area had to be reduced. Attention was focused in particular upon the aged, since they were the most visible beneficiaries of social assistance. It was assumed that the number of aged was growing rapidly and that poverty, dependency, and infirmity were becoming steadily more widespread among them. In response, the government decided that it had to abdicate much of its responsibility for the care of aged people. Instead, it was argued, families would have to bear a larger portion of the burden of providing for the elderly. This course of action was justified by using statistics and reports to demonstrate to the public that the aged had become a burden upon public funds mainly because their heartless families were "foisting them upon the government." Since few of these assumptions were based upon reality, the cost-cutting measures initiated by the government, while they created much suffering among the aged population and their families, did little to solve the economic difficulties of the province.

The following chapters investigate the condition of the aged population during the second half of the nineteenth century to determine if the aged as a population were actually as destitute, ill, or dependent as provincial officials and government reports suggested. Chapter 2 uses census material to discover who the aged of nineteenth century Ontario were, where they lived, and with whom they resided. Chapter 3 explores a variety of historical evidence to uncover the actual levels of employment, dependency, and need among this aged population. Overall, these chapters demonstrate that most aged people lived outside institutions and, despite reports of widespread destitution, were not poor, mentally or physical incapacitated, or dependent. Finally, chapters 4, 5, and 6 reveal that families did not abandon the aged. Any crisis that existed during the 1890s was the result of government policy and not the irresponsibility of Ontario's families.

An analysis of this kind sheds valuable light on the origins and accuracy of current tendencies to assume that most aged people are weak, poor, and dependent. More important, an examination of the possible motives behind the promotion of the image of the aged as weak, ill, and dependent offers insights into the basis of some current policy decisions.

Population Aging, Old-Age Dependency, and Public Policy in Historical Perspective

The current panic over the aging of the population is often assumed to be an unprecedented product of recent demographic trends, but that assumption is incorrect. The Ontario government of the 1890s had similar concerns. Analogous to the situation today, government officials assumed that in previous generations the aged population was small and that an aging population necessarily represented a unique crisis. As the following chapters shall explain, however, much of the panic nineteenth-century officials demonstrated had little to do with the actual number of old people in the province or with any real increases in the level of dependency exhibited by that group.

While many sociological writings have implied that there were few aged people in the past, historians have long debated precisely what portion of past populations were elderly and how the number of old people in any given society affected the manner in which the aged were treated and the types of assistance made available to them. The basic conclusion one gains from the bulk of the North American, French, and British historical scholarship on the topic is that, contrary to current claims, the aged have always been with us in significant numbers. Various demographic studies have demonstrated that the rate at which the aged portion of society has changed has not always been steady – it has grown slowly in some periods and rapidly in others. These studies have also shown that, even in periods when the population was aging noticeably, it is likely that the magnitude of the apparent growth in the number of aged people often had more to do with overall fertility rates and immigration trends, which produced changes in the size of other age groups in relation to the size of the aged population, than with any significant changes in the elderly population itself.

Unfortunately, precise demographic details concerning the aged are difficult to compile. Demographic statistics for past populations are often unreliable or, in some cases, non-existent. Rarely are demographic records sufficiently complete to permit exact calculations to be performed. Frequently disagreeing as to the value and meaning of most demographic information concerning past populations, historians concerned with ascertaining the exact size of the aged population in the past have reached widely divergent results. Nevertheless, most British and European demographers and historians have concluded that, whatever the difficulties in defining and identifying them, the elderly certainly were not uncommon in past centuries.[1]

The early British demographer Gregory King found that, as early as 1695, one in every ten persons was over the age of sixty.[2] This trend continued until high fertility rates changed the demographic structure in favour of children in the latter part of the eighteenth century.[3] In his study of the aged in France, Peter Stearns concurred that the old were not rare; he surmised that they were present at all levels of society and in considerable numbers.[4] This assertion was supported by the work of David Troyansky, who found that in eighteenth-century France people over the age of sixty formed as much as 15 per cent of the population over the age of twenty and up to one-quarter of the over thirty population.[5]

There is less agreement about the size of the elderly population in North America. John Demos, based on his analysis of demographic studies of various towns in seventeenth-century New England, argues that the elderly made up between 4.1 and 6.7 per cent of the total population. A higher percentage results if one considers the aged as a portion of the over-twenty population, since by far the largest segment of New England's population at this time consisted of children.[6] According to that principle, the aged formed from 8.5 to as much as 13.8 per cent of New England's adult population in the colonial era.[7] Alfred Kutzik places the aged portion of the population closer to the British standard of 10 per cent.[8] Another scholar, John B. Williamson, claims that only 6 per cent of the seventeenth-century population was at least sixty years old and 2 per cent was over the age of sixty-five.[9] Describing the situation in a different way, Demos states that at birth 44.5 per cent of the colonial population could expect to live beyond the age of sixty and that 55 per cent of the people who lived to twenty would reach old age.[10]

Other historians, such as David Hackett Fischer, argue that these figures are much too high.[11] Fischer maintains that in 1750 only one in five people lived to old age.[12] Similarly, Carole Haber hypothesizes that a mere 5 per cent of the colonial population lived beyond the age of sixty and that most people died before the age of forty.[13] These claims may be true, but only if one includes in the statistics all the infants who died. Calculations of this type are a misuse of life-expectancy tables since they almost certainly underestimate the presence of aged people in any given population.[14]

Life-expectancy charts often suggest that people in the past all died about the age of fifty, yet this was not the case. Average ages at death are pushed downwards by the massive numbers of children who died before reaching the age of five, and, for this reason, they rarely reflect the reality of most people's lives. Life-expectancy charts also provide an inflated impression of the increase in the average lifespan in recent years, since the dramatic increase in life expectancy over the last century has mainly been due to a decrease in infant deaths, not a sharp increase in adult longevity.[15] According to George Emery, it is well established that the length of life past the age of sixty-five has changed little through time.[16] The only significant change is that a larger portion of the population is reaching sixty. Consequently, Haber's figures, although they may not be inaccurate, are definitely misleading. Considering all the evidence and despite assertions to the contrary, Peter Laslett argues that, in all probability, "a fair number of people reached the higher ages."[17]

Historians such as Fischer and Demos have suggested that the degree to which old people were a common or rare element of the population determined the extent to which old people were a daily feature of life for the rest of the population. This in turn, they hypothesize, would influence how people responded to and behaved towards the aged: people would think differently about the aged if they saw old people on a daily basis rather than on only rare occasions. Haber and Fischer maintain that few people lived to old age and hence the elderly were an uncommon element in colonial society. While they draw different conclusions from this assertion, they both believe that the relative dearth of old people played a significant role in forming people's attitudes towards the aged.

Most contentions that age and the elderly were denigrated as the aged population grew depend upon the existence of a small aged population in colonial times. Yet, even if there were fewer elderly people in the past than Demos or Laslett suggest, there is no reason to assume that a small number of old people could not play an active daily role in the lives of a great many young people. In a period when 36 per cent of all families consisted of more than nine children,[18] one man living to the age of eighty could possibly have eight or nine living children, as many as forty or fifty grandchildren, and possibly as many great-grandchildren. It was also likely that several of these descendants would live in the same town, village, or settlement as this man, or nearby. Thus, it would be possible for this one old person to make an impact on the lives of as many as ninety to one hundred younger relatives. (Laurel Thatcher Ulrich recounts the case of one woman, who, at the age of eighty, had 177 grandchildren.[19]) Such figures do not include the young non-kin that aged individuals may have had contact with merely by living in close proximity to them. In short, it is clear that the elderly population did not have to be large to ensure that a majority of the people in the colonial era had daily or at least frequent contact with the aged.[20]

Population aging is a phenomenon that has occurred at various points in history. Yet the image of population aging as a "social problem" has not necessarily been related to any of these changes in the number of elderly. Instead, over the last two centuries, independent of any demographic trends, concern over the social consequences of population aging has been prevalent during some periods and virtually non-existent in others.[21] It appears that it is only when policy makers perceive the aged to be a group of mainly destitute and dependent individuals or when it is politically convenient to depict the aged as such that population aging becomes viewed as a social problem.

In England, for example, during the latter decades of the nineteenth century, the aged became a subject of intense public concern. Considerable subjective evidence was generated which supported the contention that an increasing portion of the elderly population was dependent upon public assistance. Jill Quadagno has discovered, however, that much of this evidence was in fact mere political rhetoric. In truth, the portion of the total aged population on public relief declined throughout the period.[22] This situation arose again between 1920 and 1960, when, Pat Thane reports, declining fertility rates caused concern over the "menace" of population aging.[23] Thane elaborates that throughout this period discussions of the social consequences of an aging population emphasized the elderly's dependency, loneliness, and misery even though it was admitted that most old people were not poor or alone. In both instances, social commentators were predicting that an increase in the number of old people in the population would have dire social consequences. But in neither case did the gloomy predictions of an imminent "crisis" materialize.[24]

Clearly, one of the key components of the image of the aged as a social problem is the perception that the elderly, as a population, are destitute, ill, and dependent. To varying degrees, present-day governments in Great Britain, the United States, and Ontario have tended to view the aged in these terms. As we have seen, fear of widespread old-age dependency is generally what causes governments to approach population aging as a potential crisis. Such rhetoric can be used to promote panic and convince people that otherwise unpopular measures, such as cutting services to the aged, are necessary and unavoidable. In this regard, information that promotes the idea that the old-age dependency is widespread can serve as a useful political tool.

This type of information is what Stephen Katz has labelled "alarmist demography."[25] Demographic statistics are used to convey images of impending doom which tend to create panic among the general public. The message of these reports is popular, mainly because it preys upon the public's fear of financial insecurity, and seemingly objective statistics are regularly used to "forward an ill-founded thesis."[26] The usual form of this demographic argument is "highly misleading" at best.[27] Katz, points out that "many of these 'alarmist' writers misappropriate statistical data to project the growing dependency of non-productive retirees on producing workers and then disguise such projections as inevitable facts."[28] These facts are often merely assumptions. They are accepted by the public, however, because they confirm many people's fears concerning the growing burden of public welfare. This is especially true during periods of fiscal restraint, when public opinion towards welfare harden and any increase in expenditures is seen as unacceptable.

The image of old-age dependency has had a major influence on how historians have viewed the aged. Most studies of the aged in the nineteenth century have assumed that old age was a period of poverty and dependency and have focused on explaining why this was the case. For instance, historians frequently argue that, during the onset of industrialization, deteriorating attitudes towards aged workers contributed to the poverty and dependency of the aged by drastically reducing their employment opportunities. In the same context, historians have generally assumed that there was a dramatic distinction between the ability of the aged to support themselves in an agricultural society and their prospects for survival in an industrial economy.[29] The traditional argument has been that old people were able to remain independent as long as the economy was a primarily agricultural one. Once industrialization altered this situation in the late nineteenth century, old-age dependency suddenly became widespread.

Generally, accounts of the development of retirement among the aged have rested on the assumption that retirement was rare in agricultural societies in Europe and pre-industrial America because few could afford to survive without working. As a result, older men remained employed as long as they were able to work.[30] Infirmity was the only reason to stop working and, John Demos states, it was usually the inability to work that forced people into dependency.[31] As S.J. Wright comments, the lists of the poor from the sixteenth century on "provide graphic illustration of the association between advancing years, the inability to work, and poverty."[32] Most aged people, however, asserts Judith Husbeck, were either able to support themselves until shortly before their deaths by working their land or they used their control of the land to compel their children to care for them. In this environment, argues Alfred Kutzik, the vast majority of colonial American elders required no public assistance.[33]

It appears, however, that these historians exaggerate the degree to which the aged remained independent in agricultural societies. David Thomson confutes the idea that retirement was rare in such environments, claiming that the aged were never particularly active even in the rural labour force. There is, he states, "no significant body of evidence to substantiate the claim of continued employment of the aged in the past." He explains that the aged of the eighteenth century were hardly more robust or more able to do manual labour than the aged of today. Retirement was a recognized feature of life long before the twentieth century and it was, he asserts, rare for people to continue working long after the age of sixty-five. "Retirement from work before the onset of actual physical decrepitude," he contends, "seems to have been an accepted phase of life."[34]

If the elderly were unable to support themselves because they did not work, Thomson asserts that they were maintained by their communities. Richard Smith supports this contention with evidence from early manorial courts. Retirement, he explains, "was a concept current and regularly observed."[35] In this sense, he argues that, while it did not create a social problem, old-age dependency was not uncommon in eighteenth-century England. The issue received little attention, not because the aged required no assistance, but because communities rarely questioned their obligation to provide it.[36] It is wrong, these historians argue, to assume that there must have been few poor since poor relief was not a problem.[37]

Nevertheless, historians and sociologists have long argued that industrialization and urbanization transformed the economy's occupational structure in ways that were "particularly detrimental to older members of the working class."[38] According to this argument, usually associated with modernization theory, the elderly were unable to compete in an industrial system where workers depended upon wage labour. As a result, they were unable to keep up as new machinery and a drive for higher productivity increased the pace of work in the latter decades of the century.[39] William Graebner believes that these workers were driven out of the workforce as employers attempted to improve efficiency by eliminating unproductive or less productive workers. Those aged people who remained employed, he asserts, were concentrated in low-paying clerical and subclerical occupations. He concludes that it was unemployment caused by age discrimination in the workplace which led to high levels of old-age dependency since few of these unemployed workers had access to alternate sources of income.[40] Andrew Achenbaum concludes that, while this process forced few out of the labour force prior to 1890, unemployment among the aged became significant during the next three decades.[41]

Other historians, however, have refuted these claims. Margaret Pelling, for instance, argues that in Norwich, England, an urban textile centre, evidence from as early as 1570 indicates that "older men were not radically more likely to become unemployed than younger men."[42] Similarly, Brian Gratton concludes that aged men in the United States at the end of the nineteenth century "were quite likely to remain in the labour-force."[43] Likewise, Howard Chudacoff and Tamera Hareven found consistently high employment rates for older men in Massachusetts during the final decades of the last century.[44] In Britain, meanwhile, as many as 66 per cent of the men over the aged of sixty-five were economically active in the 1890s.[45]

Even after the turn of the century, there is little evidence of advancing dependency among the aged.[46] In New York State in 1901, Sue Weiller claims, the majority of aged men were married, employed, and heads of households.[47] Many, rather than being dependants themselves, had children or other relatives who were dependent upon them.[48] Far from being destitute or decrepit, most aged people were able to care for themselves.[49] It would appear, therefore, that not only has the degree to which the aged in the distant past remained self-sufficient been overstated but that their rising poverty and dependency after 1890 has been greatly exaggerated.[50]

This may be the result of historians accepting employment as the main indicator of independence. Those without employment, it is assumed, were almost certainly left with no means of support. Many researchers assume that the ability to survive on non-employment income was rare prior to 1930, and so they have seen any decline in employment levels among the aged as a clear indication of their increasing impoverishment. Such a view rests on incorrect assumptions about the nature of retirement in past generations.

Roger Ramson and Richard Sutch state that "the history of retirement in the United States needs to be reassessed. A significant misunderstanding which has influenced much recent work on contemporary retirement is the view that retirement was uncommon before 1940."[51] Rather than having retirement forced upon them by ageist policies which removed older men from the workforce, Ramson and Sutch advance the view that retirement rates for these men were the same in 1870 as they were in 1930. They explain the discrepancy between their findings and the work of other historians by referring to the manner in which census officials recorded employment rates. Censuses, especially the one conducted in 1890, are often used to highlight the degree to which the aged were forced out of the labour force between that point and 1930. Ramson and Sutch point out, however, that the definition of employment used in these censuses provided a particularly high incidence of employment among the aged and that "a considerable number of persons who were retired or permanently disabled were reported with a gainful occupation."[52] In 1870 and 1880 people were assigned their "habitual occupation whether it is being pursued at this time or not." In 1890 anyone was included as employed if they were "in pursuit of income." People living on investment income or pensions were by this definition often counted as employed.[53]

When the employment rates for older men are recalculated by counting only those people who were actually working, the decline in the levels of employment among aged men between 1870 and 1930 disappear. The higher levels of employment previously cited were due more to changing definitions of employment than to any alteration in the actual portion of aged men who worked. Ramson and Sutch argue that, throughout this period, 64 per cent of men over the age of 60 were gainfully employed. There was, they conclude, "a significant propensity to retire at the turn of the century."[54] This would indicate that, not only were more aged people apparently able to survive while retired than was previously supposed, but there is also no indication of any decrease in their ability to support themselves through employment.[55]

As William Graebner and Andrew Achenbaum point out, many aged men, though employed, did experience what Ramson and Sutch refer to as "on the job retirement," in which they were moved, as they aged, to less demanding and lower-paid jobs. Yet, rather than seeing this phenomenon as evidence of the aged being forced out of the workforce, Ramson and Sutch argue that such occupational changes were a means of permitting the aged to retain some form of employment, and hence an income, despite a decline in their ability to perform manual labour.[56] For many, reduced employment was a transitional step on the path towards full retirement.[57]

Further evidence that retirement was a possibility for numerous aged people in late-nineteenth-century United States is offered by a study carried out by Brian Gratton and Francis Rotondo. They affirm that "economic growth engendered by industrialization had very positive effects" for many aged people and that the welfare of older people improved rather than degenerated during the industrial era.[58] At the turn of the century, many elderly people, using the earnings of their entire family, had accumulated savings and investments which provided them with an average annual retirement income of $308 a year for ten years. While these "life-cycle savings," as Ramson and Sutch refer to them, were highly dependent upon interfamilial sacrifice, family work could permit the working class to build up considerable assets with which to ward off dependency in old age. In fact, Gratton and Rotondo point out that many did more than that since the annuities produced by these savings would have provided a good standard of living for many aged people even if they no longer worked.[59] This contention is corroborated by similar information concerning the savings British workers contributed towards nineteenth-century Friendly Societies. These organizations collected funds from workers and used such to support their members in periods of illness or in their old age.[60]

In addition, Gratton and Rotondo assert that aged men were twice as likely as younger men to obtain income from sources other than employment. They also point out that, contrary to arguments concerning the declining ability of aged men to earn a living through employment, a cost-of-living survey carried out by the United States Bureau of Statistics reveals that the economic fortunes of all workers rose between 1890 and 1917 and that older men fared as well if not better than younger men in the general improvement.[61] These findings certainly suggest that, despite what government reports were saying about them, old people in the United States were far from being a helpless, dependent minority. In fact, it appears that the incidence of poverty among the aged was declining between 1870 and 1930.[62]

It is clear that the elderly were, for the most part, employed or possessed of sufficient savings or non-employment types of income to support themselves; the destitute among them were a small minority. Nevertheless, the tendency to link old age with dependency was common in nineteenth-century Ontario. Government officials regularly noted that poverty and dependency were becoming serious problems among the province's aged population. It was assumed that most people who were old were also destitute, ill, and dependent. According to the reports of inspector of prisons and public charities during the 1890s, poverty was increasingly widespread among Ontario's elderly and, consequently, growing numbers of aged people were ending their days in houses of industry, insane asylums, or local prisons. Responding to government reports, newspapers publicized the plight of the aged poor, creating in the minds of the general public the impression that most old people were living miserable lives of abject poverty.

Institutional administrators regularly lamented that most houses of industry were becoming "depositaries for the decaying and the decrepid."[63] In Toronto, for example, the number of aged people seeking admission to the House of Industry increased steadily during the latter decades of the nineteenth century. Some old people were literally dumped on the institution's doorsteps, as was one old woman who was "dropped from a wheelbarrow at the gates, by some friends."[64] By 1882 the establishment contained ninety people, "nearly all both aged and infirm."[65] A decade later, the Toronto *Empire* declared that the institution was "simply an old folk's home, a place where poor old bodies, whose lives have apparently resulted only in poverty, find shelter in their dying years."[66] Similarly, the Toronto *Mail* reported that the population of the institution was "composed of old worn out, broken down, decrepid, blind, paralysed beings who, were it not for such a place, would die in the streets of exposure."[67] Most of the people who died in such institutions were indeed elderly. Between 1866 and 1898 there was an average of ten deaths a year in Toronto's House of Industry. All but a handful of the decedents were over the age of sixty, and several were over eighty. In 1899 sixteen people died; eleven were over seventy years old.[68] To the readers of the *Globe*, it was obvious that the institution was mainly a residence for people "too old and poor to take care of themselves."[69] Similarly, insane asylum administrators complained that so many senile old people were crowding their institutions that asylums were in danger of becoming "veritable homes for incurables."[70]

Even more pitiful than the apparent hordes of aged people crowding houses of industry and insane asylums were those elderly incarcerated in jails as "vagrants." In 1897 it was reported that almost half the "criminals" held in Ontario's various county jails were merely homeless old people.[71] In some counties, jails were being used almost solely to maintain the aged poor.[72] The inspector of prisons commented in 1892 that these old people were "guilty of no crime but who on account of poverty and inability to earn for themselves a livelihood and having no friends to undertake responsibility of their care, have no other shelter." These "vagrants," he added, were committed from year to year, and frequently the aged found themselves in jail continuously for five or six years.[73]

Jails, being intended as a punishment for criminals, not as homes for the elderly poor, merely provided these old people with a cell. Poor old people were confined together with genuine criminals and the jailers rarely had any knowledge of how to care for the aged. Consequently, newspapers reported, the elderly received no care in jails and some observers felt that once committed the old were treated "worse than criminals."[74] Inside a jail, the aged were prisoners, their lives controlled entirely by prison routine and the jail-keeper. As well, conditions in nineteenth-century jails were often "squalid and inhumane."[75] One old man, for instance, arrived at the Rockwood Asylum from the Brockville jail. His eyes were cut, his face and neck were bruised and his clothes were "full of vermin."[76]

As a result of the horrid environment within some county jails, many feeble old prisoners suffered from depression and mental trauma while incarcerated. Insane asylum reports verify that people who were reportedly sane when they entered a jail suffered from attacks of "mania" or were "put off base" while confined.[77] In other instances, deaths of aged people could be directly attributed to the adverse conditions within jails. The Prisoner's Aid Association of Canada publicized the plight of aged prisoners by describing the case of one eighty-five-year-old woman named Margaret, who died in the Whitby jail in 1894. An inquest concluded that "the deprivation of her liberty, and the loss of society unhinged her reason and her constitution broke down under the strain."[78]

Together these government statements and newspaper reports helped inform the public that the number of aged poor in the province was growing. This in turn created the impression that destitution, dependence, and infirmity were widespread among Ontario's aged. By virtue of their sheer numbers, the aged poor came to dominate the public's understanding of who the aged were and how they lived. It was commonly understood that "the predominance of the aged in Almshouses is a sign of their increasing dependency,"[79] and at the same time it was widely believed that the average elderly person was a likely candidate for pauperism. One MP asserted in the House of Commons that many Canadians "spend their declining years in penury and abject dependence upon others."[80] Social workers attempting to secure assistance for these destitute old people emphasized their need and dependency to the degree that they, too, helped create in the minds of the general public the understanding that "old age, merely by that name, is a synonym for poverty."[81]

As well as being poor, the aged persons found in institutions, asylums, and county jails were usually feeble, infirm, or senile. This encouraged the idea that physical and mental incapacity were also necessary attributes of old age. Medical journals and various social commentators regularly equated old age with illness, infirmity, and senility to the point that old age itself became defined as a disease. The physical and mental weakness of the aged, it was assumed, made it impossible for elderly people to be anything but completely dependent.[82] Similar to the situation today, newspapers, public commentary, and official reports left the impression that both the financial and the physical dependency of the old were rapidly expanding and that they would continue to expand at an ever increasing rate. A major social crisis was predicted.

This crisis was frequently blamed on families. Government officials argued that the rising number of old people in institutions was largely a result of families refusing to care for their dependent elderly members. Old people were being "foisted upon the government" because their families were deciding in ever increasing numbers to transfer the burden of their care "from the home to the state."[83] It was disgraceful, one asylum official reported, "to see how many so-called Christians look upon parents in such a helpless condition as encumbrances and are prepared to commit these harmless dements to an asylum simply to get rid of them."[84] The general impression, therefore, was that during the 1890s the aged population of Ontario was largely made up of miserable, destitute people who were infirm, senile, and helpless. Their families refused to care for them and, as a result, these poor old people were mainly found in houses of industry, insane asylums, or county jails.

It is clear, however, that the poverty and dependency as well as the physical and mental incapacity of the aged population were greatly exaggerated. As Carole Haber explains, the percentage of inmates in public institutions who were elderly did not reveal that the old as a group were impoverished. By arguing that increases in the size of the aged population inside institutions reflected a rising incidence of old-age dependency, officials and social commentators were confusing the growth in the absolute numbers of old people in houses of industry or refuge with the unchanging portion of the aged population who were institutionalized.[85] Nevertheless, the perception of the aged as a largely dependent population persisted and has survived to this day.

Home and Family: A Demographic Profile of the Aged in Nineteenth-Century Ontario: Brockville, 1851–1901

Any investigation of the social, physical, and economic circumstances of the aged must begin with the issue of where and with whom the aged lived. In Canada, however, little is known about the composition of the elderly population in the nineteenth century. Several studies have charted the growth of the elderly population since 1900, but it has generally been accepted that prior to this date there was only a small population of old people in Canada and that their numbers remained fairly stable. Also, since major changes in the position of the elderly in society have occurred only in recent decades,[1] some scholars have assumed that demographic changes were absent in previous periods.[2]

Historians and demographers have used census figures only to calculate the total number of aged people in any given decade of the nineteenth century. Few studies have attempted to study the growth of Canada's or Ontario's nineteenth-century elderly population over time, or to chart changes that occurred in the composition of this group during the last half of that century. Aside from some rather sparse details, almost nothing is known about who the aged in nineteenth-century Ontario were, how they lived, or with whom they resided. To answer these questions one must use census data, one of the few sources available for such a study. Rather than merely counting the aged population, however, this analysis employs census material to locate aged households and to analyse their structure as well as any changes in their composition which occurred between 1851 and 1901.

While census figures provide the only source with which to study changes in the province's aged population over time, there are problems associated with using this information. As an indicator of how many people were over the age of sixty, census data provides no more than a close approximation of the actual size of the population. For instance, the "population by age" statistics given in each census were not always divided into comparable age groups; in certain years the population was grouped into five-year age cohorts, such as sixty to sixty-five years, and in other years ten-year age groupings were used. In addition, these ten-year groupings could run from sixty to seventy, sixty to sixty-nine, or sixty-one to seventy-one. This makes it impossible to compare the figures from decade to decade with any precision. It is also evident that in the early census reports the population was under-enumerated. Nevertheless, the aggregate census figures do provide a general indication of the major trends and demographic patterns in the composition of the province's aged population and the degree to which population aging was a genuine cause for concern among politicians, policy makers, and the general public.

There is no doubt that the population was aging during the latter half of the nineteenth century. In Canada West (Ontario) in 1851 there were 29,533 persons over the age of sixty and they formed 3 per cent of the population. Ten years later, the 55,968 people over sixty constituted 4 per cent of the population. By 1871 there were almost 75,000 aged people in Ontario comprising 4.6 per cent of the total population. This number rose to 117,791 persons or 6.1 per cent of the population in 1881 and 152,488 people or 7.2 per cent of the population in 1891. By 1901 there were 182,735 people, or 8.4 per cent of the total population of Ontario, who were over the age of sixty.[3]

These figures also reveal, however, that concern over population aging did not necessarily depend upon the actual rate at which the elderly population was increasing. After 1881, for instance, though Ontario's aged population was increasing in number, it was growing at a steadily slower rate. Even in absolute numbers, fewer additional people were added to the aged population in each of three final decades of the nineteenth century. The aged population increased at a rate of 46.8 per cent between 1851 and 1861, and 36.3 per cent between 1871 and 1881. After that date the rate of growth fell to 22.7 per cent during the 1880s and 16.6 per cent between 1891 and 1901. In absolute numbers the aged population increased by 42,791 people in the 1870s, 34,697 during the 1880s, and only 30,247 between 1891 and 1901. Yet it was during this last decade that the size of the aged population came to be perceived as a social problem by the Ontario government. In other words, concern about the growth of the aged population developed after that growth had begun to slow down.[4] (See Figure 1.)

This does not mean that the aged were rare. In comparison to the current size of the elderly population, the nineteenth-century figures seem low. However, the increase in the portion of the population over the age of sixty that occurred during the twentieth century was not entirely attributable to growth in the numbers of old people. It also re-

Figure 1
The aged as a percentage of the total population of Ontario compared to the rate of
growth of the aged population, 1861–1901

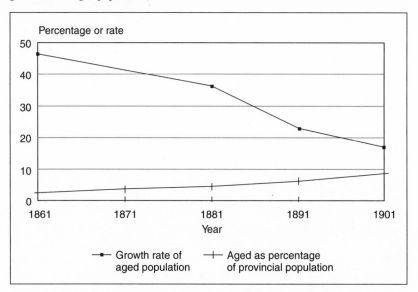

flected the significant decline in the crude birth rate.[5] Declining
fertility rates and the shrinking of the size of the population under the
age of twenty automatically increase the portion of the population
who are aged, even if the actual number of people in this group does
not grow.

In 1851 and even 1861, Canada West was, to a large degree, still a
frontier community. The population of such regions is often composed of recent settlers who tend to be young. Moreover, in the 1830s
and 1840s the region experienced massive immigration, which further
increased the number of younger people in the population. A large
population of young adults also produces a large quantity of children.
In 1851, 56.8 per cent of the total population of Canada West was
under the age of twenty. Even as late as 1901, children made up 42
per cent of the total population of the province.[6] These figures are
similar to those discovered by American historians for the colonial
period. In both regions, the high numbers of children tended to dis-
tort population figures, making the aged population appear smaller
than it was.[7]

The current aged population appears larger in comparison to that of
the colonial period or the early nineteenth century mainly because there
are far fewer children in the population today. Consequently, it is advis-

able to eliminate children from the calculations[8] before comparing the size of the aged population of the last century with that of today. By focusing only on what portion of the adult population (those people over the aged of twenty) was over sixty, a more accurate picture of how common the elderly were among the population can be gained.

In 1851, 7.2 per cent of the over-twenty population was elderly. This percentage rose to almost 10 per cent in 1861 and 10.32 per cent in 1871. The elderly formed over 13 per cent of the adult population in 1891 and by 1901 almost 17 per cent of all people over the age of twenty were elderly.[9] These statistics, which are comparable to the findings of David Troyansky for eighteenth-century France and David Thomson for eighteenth- and nineteenth-century England,[10] indicate that in 1851 every fourteenth adult person was over the age of sixty but by 1901 every sixth adult was aged. In 1901 one was more than twice as likely to encounter elderly people among the population as forty years earlier.

The elderly, therefore, were not an insignificant minority of the population of Upper Canada in 1851, and over the course of the latter half of the century, while their numbers may not have grown as fast as some reports suggested, they became increasingly visible.

Of course, as Peter Laslett points out, numbers and statistics, in and of themselves, are inadequate to describe the lives of the people being counted.[11] The aggregate figures given above provide a general impression of how numerous the elderly were in Ontario during the nineteenth century and how the size of this population grew. They offer no information on other vital questions concerning where and with whom the aged lived or what changes occurred within the aged population itself. While investigating these questions on a province-wide scale would require a massive research effort, it is possible to obtain a profile of the aged in one community. No single community can represent the specific situation in all locations across the province; every village and town was unique in some respect. Yet there were towns that were not strikingly atypical and these can be regarded as representative of others.

Brockville, in Leeds County, is one such community. The town is large enough to provide a sample that is of an adequate size to study but not unmanageable. Furthermore, economically, socially, and demographically, Brockville was unexceptional.[12] It was a thriving, medium sized town at a time when the vast majority of Ontario's people lived in or near similar towns.[13] The elderly population in Brockville during the nineteenth century was in all probability not unlike the aged portion of most of Ontario's towns and villages. At the very least, therefore, a study of Brockville's aged population between 1851 and 1901 provides an example of general demographic trends and living arrangements among the aged in nineteenth-century Ontario.

The census district of Brockville included the town and the surrounding rural areas. For the purposes of this study, a detailed analysis was carried out only on the town; a sampling of the information on the rural areas produced results that were similar to those for Brockville. This is not to argue that the rural experience of the aged was identical to that of the elderly in towns. The differences noted in this one case, however, did not appear significant enough to warrant a comparative study. In addition, a sample, which included the Frontenac and Cataraqui wards of Kingston and the central ward of St Catharines, was taken from the 1901 census to allow a comparison of the demographic profile of Brockville at the turn of the century with that of other regions of the province. For the most part, these results confirmed the initial impression that the situation in Brockville was not unlike the general situation across the province.

The information required to piece together a profile of Brockville's aged population is found in the manuscript census data and the printed census material. The reports of 1851, 1891, and 1901 have been chosen for this study. Although, in theory, these census reports provide a listing of every person who lived in Brockville in the years mentioned, there are several problems with them.[14] The printed census material offers population totals and breakdowns of the population by age group. Since these totals were obtained from the manuscript census data, the aggregate figures in the printed census material should duplicate the results obtained by totalling the names in the manuscript census. This, however, is not the case. In 1851, for example, the printed census states that there were 105 people over the age of sixty in the town. Unfortunately, the census report from one of the three sections of the town is missing from the manuscript census. Hence, it is possible to locate only two-thirds of the total households. In the printed census for 1891, the total population of the census district of Brockville, which was much larger than the town itself, is given as 15,853 people. Yet the breakdown of that population into age groups totals 17,333 people.

It is also likely that in both censuses several people did not report their correct age. Many people may not have known their age, while others, especially older people, may have purposely deceived the census takers, either out of spite or because of a wish to keep their actual age private. As the Brockville *Recorder* reported in 1851, the women of the community were quite indignant when the receiver general announced that they would have to report their precise age to the enumerators. It was expected that few would comply with this request.[15]

For these reasons, the census data for Brockville in both 1851 and 1891 are not completely reliable. The 1901 census is far more accurate than any of the earlier censuses, but it is likely that it, too, contains errors, omissions, and incomplete data. Nevertheless, while a detailed and precise investigation of the aged population of Brockville in either 1851 or 1901 is not possible, the information is sufficient to describe the basic characteristics of the aged population and to assess which living arrangements were most common for this group. The specific numbers, percentages, and averages may not be completely accurate, but the trends and characteristics they portray are certainly representative of the true state of the aged population of Brockville.

An examination of changes in the size, composition, and living arrangements of Brockville's aged population highlights three issues concerning the aged in nineteenth-century Ontario and the government's response to them. Between 1851 and 1901, the elderly population in Brockville increased in both actual numbers and as a portion of the population. By 1901 a larger number of these people were very old and more of them were in categories social historians have normally associated with poverty and dependency, such as widows and never-married individuals. However, the bulk of these changes occurred in the decades prior to 1891. During the 1890s, when concerns about the number of aged people in the population were being expressed, the rate of growth of the aged population was actually slowing down.[16] Consequently, the alarming trends that officials predicted never materialized.

In addition, despite claims that a larger portion of these aged people were becoming dependent throughout this period, the majority of the elderly people in Brockville headed their own household or were married to a household head. The number of aged people who lived with children or kin increased both in absolute numbers and as a portion of the total aged population. Regardless of official statements concerning the role of the family in the care of the aged, the census data from Brockville indicates that, rather than shirking their responsibilities towards the aged, Ontario's families became more, not less, significant to the aged over the course of the nineteenth century.

GENERAL DEMOGRAPHICS

According to the printed census of 1851, Brockville contained 3,236 residents. It is possible to locate only 1,916, or 60 per cent, of these people in the manuscript census, since records exist for the east and west wards only. The total number of aged in the town is given as 105 in the printed census; the manuscript census includes 73, or 70 per cent, of these people. The figures from the surviving manuscript census will be those used to represent the town of Brockville in 1851. In total, 3.8 per cent of the population of the town was aged and these elderly people were dispersed among 18.5 per cent of the community's households. These people were on average sixty-five years old.[17]

By 1891 the population of the town had risen to 8,791 people, distributed among 1,602 households. The town's 498 aged citizens resided in 385 households. Thus, the aged were found in 24 per cent of the households and formed 5.4 per cent of the total population. Ten years later, in 1901, Brockville's 670 aged people made up 6.4 per cent of Brockville's population. In the fifty years between 1851 and 1901, then, the aged population grew substantially, not only in actual numbers but as a portion of the population. The result was that as the nineteenth century progressed, at least in Brockville, old people were present in more households and were a common feature of daily life for an increasingly larger segment of the population. It does not seem that the size of Brockville's aged population was in anyway exceptional. In fact, in Kingston and St Catharines in 1901, the aged represented an even larger segment of the total population than they did in Brockville. In the two largest wards in Kingston, Frontenac and Cataraqui, the aged made up, respectively, 6.3 and 7.6 per cent of the population. In St Catharines, elderly people accounted for over 8 per cent of the population.

As well as becoming more numerous, the elderly were older in 1891 than they had been in 1851. While their average age was 65.6 years in 1851, by 1891 it had risen to sixty-eight. The aging of the population becomes even more obvious when one considers that in 1851 there were only three people over the age of eighty while in 1891 over 10 per cent of the aged population was at least eighty years old. Meanwhile, 36.5 per cent of the aged population was at least seventy years old.

Despite numerous reports of the increase in the numbers of very aged people in the population during the 1890s, between 1891 and 1901 there was actually no change in the percentage of the aged population who were very old. About 10 per cent were over eighty and 36 per cent were over the aged of seventy. In Kingston and St Catharines the very old formed a slightly smaller portion of the aged population; people over the age of eighty formed less than 8 per cent of the total sample, and approximately one-third of the elderly were over seventy. This population did grow in absolute numbers, but, as will be demonstrated, the number of children and kin caring for these people also grew.

Over the last half of the nineteenth century, the aged population changed not only in size and age but also in composition: the main change being that women, especially widows, became more common.

Men formed the majority of the population at mid-century; by 1901 women dominated. In 1851 the elderly population of Brockville consisted of forty-three males and only thirty females. In 1891, however, women outnumbered men, forming 52 per cent of the population. Over the next decade the gender balance remained stable, with 53 per cent of the aged population being female. Similarly, in Kingston, women formed 54 per cent of the aged people in Frontenac and Cataraqui wards in 1901, while they constituted over 56 per cent of the sample from St Catharines. This suggests that more women were living longer, an impression confirmed by overall mortality trends.[18] Studies of mortality rates in Toronto and England have concluded that there was a disproportionately rapid fall in female deaths over the nineteenth century.[19] This trend would, in turn, have had an impact on the marital status of aged people.

If more women were living longer, fewer wives would pre-decease their husbands. This would be indicated by a decrease in the number of widowers and a corresponding increase in the numbers of both widows and married men. Such is indeed what occurred in Brockville. Between 1851 and 1901 the portion of widowed men among the aged population fell from 16.4 to only 8.8 per cent. During the same period widows, who formed 21.9 per cent of the population in 1851, came to comprise one-third of the town's aged. There was also a steady increase in the number of married women; they formed 16.4 per cent of the population in 1851, 18 per cent in 1891, and 20 per cent by 1901. The 1901 census for Kingston and St Catharines reveals a similar breakdown of the aged population by marital status. (See Figure 2.)

The fact that more women were living to old age is also suggested by changes that occurred in the age differential between elderly husbands and wives between 1851 and 1901. In 1851 most aged men were wed to much younger women. While the average age of these men was sixty-six years, the average age of their wives was fifty-two. Almost three-quarters of the wives were at least ten years younger than their husbands. In at least two cases, twenty-six-year-old women were married to sixty-five-year-old men. Several of these were probably second marriages for the man.[20]

In both 1891 and 1901 fewer men were married to such young spouses. On average, there was only an eight-year difference between husbands and wives. The shrinking age gap among older couples becomes even more apparent if the exceptional marriages are eliminated from the total. When calculations are performed using the 80 per cent of the marriages in which there was less than twelve years between the spouses, the average age difference in 1891 is reduced to 5.6 years. There were still some men who married much younger women.

Figure 2
Widows and widowers, 1851 and 1901

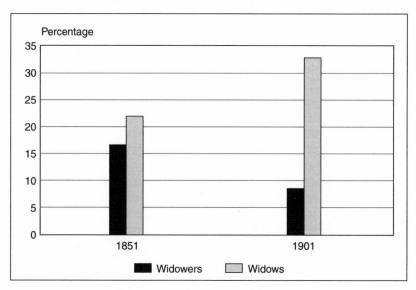

William Robinson, for instance, aged sixty, lived with his thirty-year-old wife Elizabeth, while eighty-year-old Joseph Thompson was married to a forty-year-old woman. Yet, unlike 1851, when age differences of at least ten years were the rule, such marriages were definitely exceptional in 1891. Then, only one in five aged men were involved in unions with a ten-year age gap.

This evidence, combined with the increase in the number of married aged women, suggests that fewer wives were dying young. That fact in turn meant that fewer older men would have been required to take a second and usually younger wife. It would also mean that the wives of aged men would in general be older themselves. In 1891 the average age of older men's wives was sixty years, which was eight years older than the average in 1851. The longer that women lived, the more likely they were to outlive their husbands. This would account for the rise in the population of widowed women.

The increase in number of aged women not only resulted in a rise in the ages of the spouses of aged men but was also at least partially responsible for significant alterations in the living arrangements and family structure of the aged population as a whole. By 1891, where and with whom the aged lived, the relationship they had with these people, and the way the aged fit into the community had all been altered.

HOUSEHOLDS

Among the households containing aged people, the most common type in Brockville in 1851, 1891, and 1901 was one headed by a male, between the ages of sixty-five and sixty-eight, who lived with a wife aged between fifty and sixty years and three or four unmarried children between the ages of fifteen and thirty-three.[21] While this broad portrait of the most common group of aged persons in Brockville implies that little changed among the elderly population during the latter half of the nineteenth century, a great deal more change occurred than these averages would indicate. To reach a true understanding of how the aged population of 1901 differed from that of fifty years earlier, it is necessary to look beyond average traits and examine the aged population in detail.

Despite claims that the aged were becoming an increasingly dependent population, in every Brockville census schedule examined the vast majority of the aged lived independently and maintained their own homes. In fact, in each census year, it was more common to find aged people heading households including other dependent people, usually their children, than to locate aged people living as dependants in the homes of others. In 1851, 71.2 per cent of the households that contained an aged person, or 13.2 per cent of the total households in Brockville, were headed by an aged person. Most of these household heads (83 per cent) were male and over half of these men were married, while the remainder were almost all widowers. With one exception, all female household heads were widows.

In 1901, as in 1851, the majority of the aged people in Brockville were heads of their own households. Almost three-quarters of the homes in which an old person resided were headed by a person who was at least sixty years old. As in 1851, the bulk of these households heads (69 per cent) were men in their mid-sixties. However, a greater percentage of these male households heads were married (86 per cent), while the rest were mainly widowers. There were also more households (31 per cent) headed by women. As in 1851, these women were mainly widows in their mid-sixties (94 per cent). Such changes again reflect the increasing number of elderly women in the population. There were more households headed by women and more widows, mainly because more women were living longer and outliving their husbands. There were also more married men, because more of their wives were living longer.

In all three census reports, the majority of aged household heads had children living with them. In 1851, however, there was a clear distinction between both the number and the ages of the children in the homes of married household heads and those in the homes of widowed individuals. Since many of the married-male aged household heads in Brockville in 1851 had much younger spouses, it is not surprising that several of these elderly men also had children (four on average) who were fairly young, the average age being 15.5 years. Widowed people, on the other hand, usually had only one or sometimes two children living with them and these children were generally unmarried adults, although four households contained widowed children and some grandchildren. The average age of the children in the home of widowed individuals was twenty-two years.

By 1891 the reduction in the age differential between married men and women and the decline in the number of May-December marriages had altered the family structure of Brockville's aged men. As in 1851, the majority (67.8 per cent) of the aged household heads lived with children. However, the children in these households were much older than the children had been forty years earlier. As well, there was no longer any distinction between the age and number of children in the homes of married-male household heads and those in the homes of widows. This was mainly because there was no longer a difference between the ages of the wives of married men and the ages of widows. Hence, 70 per cent of the households headed by an aged person who lived with children, or half of all households headed by an aged person, contained only adult children, two on average. The average age of all adult children in these homes was 28.8 years. A typical example of this was Elizabeth Millroy, a seventy-year-old widow, who lived with her three children, Mary, aged twenty-nine, Rebecca, twenty-two, and John, thirty-two. All were single and employed.

Households with younger children usually contained only one or two children under the age of eighteen and others who were older. Few homes headed by an aged person contained only young children. The household of sixty-seven-year-old Peter Poulin, a locomotive engineer, and his wife, Nellie, aged sixty-two, was not unusual. The couple lived with seven children: Peter, thirty-six, Mary, twenty-nine, Delli, twenty-five, Adele, twenty-six, Levi, twenty-four, Adolphus, twenty-two, and one younger child, Eva, aged fourteen. Rather than containing young dependent children, as they did in 1851, aged households in 1891 included children who were often employed and did not require a great degree of parental care. In those households where there was a child who may have required care, there were other adult siblings around who could assist.

Almost three-quarters of the adult children living in the homes of their aged parents in 1891 were daughters, most of whom were single and over the age of twenty-five, which was the age at which most

women married in nineteenth-century Ontario.[22] The large number of
unmarried daughters in these homes was probably due to a rising rate
of celibacy among women in Ontario during the latter quarter of the
nineteenth century. Peter Ward explains that this trend can be attributed to several factors, the main one being that the ratio of single men
to women became less favourable over the course of the century. Also,
as the Brockville *Recorder* stated in 1892, "The failure of young men
to marry has compelled hundreds of thousands of young women to
earn an independent living. It is ... a grave social problem."[23] Ward ad-
mits, however, that no one factor alone can sufficiently explain why
many women in late-Victorian Ontario never married. Also, when
Ward calculates changes in the marriage market for women, he examines the sex ratios only for younger single people. Ward probably un-
derestimates the degree to which the number of available men declined
between 1851 and 1891 for he does not include in his calculations the
effect of increased female longevity. In 1851 many older men would
find themselves widowed and would, as a result, remarry, usually to a
younger woman. By 1891, given the declining death rates of married
women, fewer marriages were terminated by the death of the wife, and
hence fewer older men were in need of a second, and usually younger,
wife.

While some women remained single because they could not find a
husband, Ruth Freeman and Patricia Klaus mention that in late-Victorian England and North America many women preferred not to marry
because they felt single women could lead happier, freer lives.[24] The
census data on aged households in Brockville supports this claim by
suggesting one reason why remaining single became a viable option for
women during this period: in contrast to many of their predecessors in
earlier decades, they had a place to live.

In the middle decades of the nineteenth century, fewer people lived
beyond the age of sixty. Hence, as Ellen Gee explains, many women expected that before they reached the age of thirty their parents would be
dead.[25] Once a woman's parents were dead she had few options. Either
she married or lived as a spinster aunt in the home of a relative, since it
was rarely acceptable, or financially possible, for a single woman to
live alone.[26] In 1891, however, more parents were living longer. A
woman who did not wish to marry, or who could not marry, had the
option of remaining in the home of her aged parents. Some of these
daughters chose to remain at home to care for feeble or incapacitated
parents because they felt it was their duty. One remembered that "as a
dutiful daughter, I simply did my job – I accepted the standard of the
times that daughters belonged to their families."[27] Other women may
have been forced to remain at home by overbearing parents or sib-

lings.[28] In most circumstances, however, this arrangement quite likely offered many women a degree of freedom and financial security they could have never experienced in the home of a husband or as lone women in a nineteenth-century town. Whatever the reason, Marvin McInnis notes that, during the latter decades of the nineteenth century, remarkably large numbers of young women remained in their parental homes and did so to surprisingly advanced ages.[29]

These trends gained strength during the 1890s. By 1901 even more households headed by an aged person contained children (69.5 per cent), a greater percentage of these households (over 80 per cent) contained only adult offspring whose average age was close to thirty years, and more of these children (90 per cent) were female, the majority of whom (69 per cent) were single. Some aged parents housed married children and many others sheltered widowed daughters or sons, but the most common child living with aged parents was an unmarried adult daughter. This was particularly true if the parent was a widow. As in Brockville in 1901, single adult daughters were a common feature in the homes of aged people in Kingston and St Catharines.

The fact that after 1891 aged couples had mainly adult children living with them created a situation in which households headed by aged people became distinct from the majority of the households in Brockville. In 1851 over half the population of Brockville consisted of children under the age of eighteen. Almost every household in the town contained young children. In this regard, an old man with a young wife and young children was the head of a family which was not unlike the majority of the other families. Forty years later, although most aged households still contained offspring, few of these were young. Although the "empty nest syndrome" had not yet affected many aged households,[30] the structure of these aged households with only adult children was different from that of the majority of the households of the era, which still contained mainly young children. Over the course of the century, then, households headed by aged individuals became more atypical and hence more segregated from the rest of the households than they had been earlier in the century. This may have helped contribute to the idea of old age as a distinct phase of life. At the very least, it may have made it easier for people to believe government statements concerning the condition of the aged population. The segregation of the elderly possibly resulted in the general populace having less contact with them and therefore less knowledge about or understanding of their real living conditions.

In both 1851 and 1891, household heads who did not live with children generally lived alone, either as a single person or a couple.[31] While 25.9 per cent of all aged household heads lived alone in 1891, only 21

per cent of them did so ten years later. This reduction seemingly contradicts arguments that the aged were being increasingly left alone to fend
for themselves. Though people who did not live with their children
were more likely to have unrelated lodgers in their home, few aged people had other kin or non-kin aside from domestics and servants living
with them.[32] Such people were not necessarily isolated or lonely, however, for it appears that many aged people who did not live with their
children lived near them. Census data does not allow one to determine
the relationship of one household head to another, but the presence of
neighbours with the same last name as an elderly couple and in the correct age group to have been their children does suggest that many aged
couples lived close enough to one or more of their children to ensure
that they received the care they needed even though they lived alone.
An examination of the wills of those aged people found in the 1891
census indicates that most of them did indeed have offspring living in
Brockville. As well, many wills mention siblings, nieces, and nephews
who lived nearby and "showed affection" to their aged kin.[33]

The number of aged people in need of some form of either physical
or financial assistance probably increased between 1851 and 1901. We
do not really know how many people comprised the dependent portion
of the aged population. The only estimate available is the number of
persons who lived in the home of another. Yet this calculation, used by
researchers such as Howard Chudacoff and Tamera Hareven, is problematic. Living with another person does not necessarily indicate either
physical or financial dependency or need.[34] Relying on census data
alone, one can assume only that those aged people, aside from wives,
who lived in the homes of others, or non-heads, as they will be called
from this point, were more likely than aged household heads to require
assistance of some form.

Less than one-third (29 per cent) of the aged population of Brockville in 1851 lived as a non-head in the home of another person. The
bulk of them (90 per cent) were widowed and most (60 per cent) were
female. They were generally older than household heads, being an average of sixty-seven years old, and almost all lived with sons[35] or sons-in-
law.[36] The children who sheltered their parents were usually married
and had children of their own.

There was a marked increase in the size of the non-head aged population between 1851 and 1891: in 1851 they formed less than 1 per
cent of the total population of the town, but by 1891 almost 3 per cent
of the community fell into this group. During the next ten years, however, the portion of Brockville's non-head aged population shrank to
less than 2 per cent. In the sampled sections of Kingston and St Catharines, an equivalent portion of the total population, 1.9 and 2.1 per

cent respectively, belonged to this group in 1901. It is possible that there were fewer aged people living in the homes of others because their families had sent them away to institutions, yet, as shall be demonstrated later, the proportion of the aged population being institutionalized during this period remained stable. A more likely hypothesis is that the presence of unmarried adult daughters in the homes of their elderly parents encouraged some aged people to retain headship of their household. If these daughters were not present, and fewer were in 1851, many aged people would have moved in with married children instead of retaining their own household. In this manner, as the number of adult offspring who chose to remain in the home of their parents grew, the size of the non-head aged population shrank.

As in 1851, the majority of the non-head aged people in 1891 were widows. They tended to be a few years older than the non-heads had been forty years earlier, with an average age of seventy. The aged men who lived in the homes of other people were generally even older than the women, being on average seventy-six years old, and they were often married and lived together with their wives. Females were even more common among this group in 1901, forming 66 per cent of the dependent population. Three-quarters of these women were widows while the remainder were single. Over half were more than seventy years old, and another quarter were over eighty.

In 1891 the majority (65 per cent) of the these elderly non-heads lived with their children, as they had in 1851. By 1901 the portion of dependent aged people living with their children had dropped to 52.1 per cent, but, as mentioned, this may have been due to the increase in the numbers of unmarried daughters who lived with their parents. Also, while the portion of dependants living with children decreased, there was a corresponding increase in the portion who lived with other kin. Only 3 per cent of the aged dependants were listed as living with kin in 1891, whereas 19 per cent lived with siblings, nieces, or nephews in 1901.

This change reflects the increase in the portion of single aged people who had no children with whom to live.[37] As will be discussed below, however, the degree of change between 1891 and 1901 may have been exaggerated. As well, many married people, approximately 15 per cent of all couples at the turn of the century, remained childless.[38] Ellen Gee notes, too, that there was a steady decline in the number of children born to each married couple. This declining birth rate was, in fact, the outstanding feature of demographic change in Canada in the latter half of the nineteenth century. Meanwhile, child mortality rates remained high. Jane Synge reports that the combination of these trends resulted in a large number of aged people with no surviving children.[39] It is clear, however, that in the absence of children other kin were willing to shelter an aged relative. When all family members are considered, a total of 67 per cent of the aged non-heads in Brockville lived with a relative in 1891, while 71 per cent lived with a family member in 1901. The situation in both Kingston and St Catharines was comparable. In 1901 a total of 67.5 per cent of all aged non-heads located in these communities lived with a family member, 80 per cent of these relatives being adult children. These figures demonstrate that relatives played a not insignificant role in the lives of the aged and that their role may very well have increased in importance over the last decade of the nineteenth century.

A total of 36.4 per cent of the dependent aged in Brockville in 1891 were listed as lodgers in the homes of an unrelated individual. It is possible that several of these people were actually related to the household head, most probably as parents-in-law, but were not listed as such. This possibility gains strength when the information from 1891 is compared to the 1901 census data, which listed family relationships more accurately. By then, the percentage of lodgers and boarders among the aged had declined to 17.4 per cent, a reduction of more than 50 per cent. Either many more relatives began sheltering their aged family members between 1891 and 1901, which would contradict everything the government was saying about a decline in familial responsibility for the aged, or many of the lodgers listed in 1891 were in fact related to the household head. Whatever the case, these figures place in doubt any statements concerning a lack of familial support for the aged.

CONCLUSION

Despite their approximate nature, the figures set out in this chapter reveal the main trends in the composition and living arrangements of Brockville's aged population over the last half of the nineteenth century. Above all, they present a picture of the aged that often contradicts much of what was being said about them in newspaper articles and by government officials. Despite claims about the prevalence of dependency among the aged, in 1901 the aged of Brockville were more, not less, likely to be living independently and heading their own households than they were in 1891 or 1851. Also, while institutional officials reported that decreasing amounts of care were being given to the elderly by their families, in fact adult children became more rather than less common in the homes of the aged, either living as dependants in their parents' homes or housing their parents in their own homes. In addition, relatives other than children became more significant to the dependent aged as more old people were found in the homes of siblings, nieces, or nephews. Contrary to reports of a population of impoverished, abandoned, and helpless old people, aged people who lived alone were exceptional in Brockville throughout the nineteenth century. This situation resembles that found in the United States, where Tamera Hareven discovered that throughout the nineteenth century the nuclear family was the major locus of support for the aged[40] and that the incidents of family care increased, not decreased, in the 1890s.

Census data concerning where and with whom people lived provides only a partial impression of the level of dependency or need among the aged population. A detailed survey of the income as well as the physical and mental capacities of these people is required to assess just how dependent or independent the elderly were during the 1890s. It is to this issue that we now turn.

Census data doesn't include homeless.

CHAPTER THREE

Dependency, Employment, and Need among Ontario's Aged: Perception and Reality

Until recently, most literature on the history of the aged, accepting the general argument of government reports, has focused on their poverty and dependency.[1] This has certainly been true of Canadian historical writing on the subject. Richard Deaton, for instance, sums up the basic premise of most historical work on the aged when he asserts that "in British North America the condition of the elderly has been characterized by their continuous impoverishment from at least the early nineteenth-century."[2]

In Canada, it has only been in the last two decades that historians have begun to study the aged, and, despite growing interest in the subject and the overall high quality of writing in the field, the number of works concentrating specifically on the aged remains small. As well, Canadian historians have focused on only one segment of the elderly population, the aged poor. Studies of the elderly have been almost exclusively concerned with those aged people who required public relief, institutional care, or some other form of support from either the state or their families.[3] Almost without exception, therefore, the historical literature asserts that Canadians' twilight years were ones "of economic and physical dependence" and that these conditions were the product of old age[4]; indeed, it appears to proceed from the assumption that to be old was to be poor. The assumption of poverty has been so strong that few attempts have been made to determine exactly what portion of the aged population was actually poor.

There are several possible explanations as to why historians have concentrated upon the aged poor. The first of these concerns the nature of the available sources. Most of the easily accessible sources pertaining to the aged are government reports. As a result, almost every article on the aged in Canada relies upon government reports, institutional records, or the records of government agencies.[5] Each of these sources, however, focus on the aged poor; government officials and institutional administrators had little reason to be concerned with those elderly people who did not require public support. More significantly, Ann Shola Orloff has argued that late-nineteenth-century governments had a vested interest in overstating the burden the aged represented to the public purse in order to gain support for fiscal-restraint policies that tended to focus on groups such as the aged poor.[6] Yet most historians have placed great faith in the documents generated by government officials and have been reluctant to question the information within them, perhaps because they began their research already convinced that the elderly in the past were an impoverished group. When the most accessible sources confirmed what historians expected would be the case, they saw little reason to look farther.

At the same time, recent scholarship in the social sciences has helped promote the current image of the elderly as a largely dependent group. As Sara Arber and Jay Ginn have explained, when the aged are mentioned by social scientists it is most frequently in reference to the burden they pose to other people.[7] Sociological literature on the family often speaks about the aged only in terms of the stress they place on intergenerational relations. Feminist scholars refer to older people only to highlight the fact that caregiving for the aged is a particularly female burden. Social-policy research, meanwhile, "welfarizes" the elderly, discussing them only in terms of their needs as recipients. It seems that Canadian historians have been influenced by this body of social-science literature. Accepting popular images that portray today's aged population as dependent and marginalized, they have turned to the past to search for the causes of this situation.

Finally, the history of old age initially emerged as a subfield of social history. One of the main goals of social historians was to rescue the anonymous, the marginalized, and the dispossessed from the realm of the historical unknown to which traditional historians had consigned them. As the significance of social history grew, studies of the elite and powerful were seen as old-fashioned. While this way of thinking may have produced a balance of knowledge in fields where much was known about the wealthy and powerful but almost nothing about the lowly and anonymous, it created an imbalance in the study of the aged. Since elites were "passé" and the poor were "de rigueur," it is arguable that interest developed in the history of the aged primarily because most of these people were regarded as poverty-stricken.

By focusing on welfare and poverty among the aged, historians have, perhaps unintentionally, helped to reinforce the association of old age and dependency.[8] They have also promoted the idea that social-welfare measures in the twentieth century rescued a population of unemployed and neglected aged people from certain destitution. Yet the truth is much different. During the 1890s there was general ignorance about the extent of destitution and need among Canada's aged; no statistical studies of the elderly were conducted in that decade and as late as 1928 Canadian officials were relying on extrapolations from a 1910 Massachusetts study.[9] The available evidence reveals, however, that contrary to common assumptions, the vast majority of elderly people in late-nineteenth-century Ontario lived independently and were capable of maintaining themselves.

One of the main problems involved in ascertaining the economic circumstances of the aged in the past is that the terms "destitution" and "dependency" are often confused and rarely precisely defined. Frequently, the words are used interchangeably and it is assumed that anyone who was destitute was also dependent and vice versa. For the purposes of this chapter, destitution shall refer to a complete lack of financial resources, while the term dependent will be used to describe those people who received financial assistance or physical support. As an examination of census reports, employment records, and other documents such as wills demonstrates, destitute people could be independent (in the sense that they refused public support) and some dependent people were far from destitute. It is also clear that people could be dependent upon others for either physical or financial support without being helpless.[10]

As mentioned earlier, sociologists and historians have frequently asserted that industrialization and urbanization, which were accelerating in Ontario during the 1890s, transformed the occupational structure in ways that were "particularly detrimental to older members of the working class."[11] In an industrial system where workers depended upon wage labour, the elderly, it is argued, were unable to compete. As Desmond Morton asserts, in the industrializing economy of late-Victorian Canada, old age was the "ultimate disaster."[12] The aged were the most likely group of any age category to experience a decline in their employment status and, as a result, the threat of poverty was never far off.[13]

Only a detailed examination of the financial resources and standard of living of Canada's aged could confirm or refute statements concerning levels of old-age dependency in nineteenth-century Canada; however no systematic investigation of the lives of average aged people in this period has been carried out.[14] Almost all historical studies dealing with the aged have been premised upon the assumption that Canada's aged, as a population, have always been needy and dependent upon others. Yet even a brief examination of the living arrangements, workforce participation, and lifestyles of Ontario's elderly in the last century provides considerable evidence that this was not the case. There is, for instance, no conclusive evidence of widespread unemployment among Ontario's elderly during the 1890s. Nor does the available census data confirm that those people who worked earned too little to survive. Furthermore, an examination of the wills of aged people indicates that even unemployed and apparently dependent aged individuals possessed assets which provided them with an adequate income. As well, evidence from newspapers, diaries, and correspondence contradicts the claim that the elderly were, for the most part, mentally or physically incapacitated. In short, the evidence that does exist supports the argument that, at the end of the last century, Ontario's aged population was composed mainly of independent, mentally capable people who either worked or supported themselves with savings or investment income.

It has been asserted that, prior to 1940 few aged people achieved the minimum level of income required for independent living.[15] In the last chapter, however, we saw that the majority of aged people in nineteenth-century Brockville, St Catharines, and Kingston were household heads, and this finding is significant if Brian Gratton is correct in his claim that "household headship provides a fairly valid and reliable measure of economic and social self-sufficiency."[16] As well, most of the aged men in these communities were employed. While a detailed examination of employment trends is beyond the scope of this chapter, a general survey of the census data reveals that as late as 1901, a decade after unemployment due to age discrimination was supposed to have had a significant effect on old men's labour-force participation, between 64 and 76 per cent of the aged men in Kingston, Brockville, and St Catharines worked. Considering that forced unemployment due to the impact of ill health was most common among men over the age of seventy, it is significant that 41 per cent of the aged men included in this survey fell into that age group. Although it has been noted that retired individuals were regularly recorded in nineteenth-century census reports as employed,[17] this was not the case with Canada's 1901 census, which included a separate category for retired people. One can assume, therefore, that all older men listed as employed in the 1901 census were active in the labour force.

The 1901 census also permits historians to calculate how much working men earned. Though these figures are most likely not entirely accurate, and many people did not reveal their income, an analysis of the incomes reported by aged men can provide at least a general indication of whether older men were earning enough to support themselves. In Kingston, St Catharines, and Brockville, approximately two-thirds of the employed older men reported their income. Some reported annual earnings as high as $2,000 and others earned as little as $90.

Reported earnings between $300 and $600 were most common. The average income in the three communities ranged between $389 and $404. There was little variation by community or even within different sections of these towns. In all three locations and in every ward studied, the average fell into this narrow range.

These figures could be vitiated by the portion of working men who did not report their income. It seems, however, that failure to report income was at least equally prevalent among those people who most likely earned more than average as it was among men who earned less. People employed as accountants, doctors, and merchants were just as likely, and possibly more likely, not to report an income as were lower-income people such as labourers, painters, or carpenters. A large portion of those men who did not report an income were "working on their own account" or self-employed. In this regard, it is significant that in his study of self-employed men in nineteenth-century Brantford, David Burley found that over one-third of the aged businessmen were among the wealthiest 20 per cent.[18] This finding certainly suggests that the average incomes of older men could be higher than the earnings recorded in the census. Also, a number of the men listed in the census would normally be considered dependent because they lived in the home of another person. In fact, however, many of these men worked and some earned considerable incomes. Consequently, even the dependent portion of the aged population may not have been destitute or totally unable to contribute towards their care or shelter.

To determine if the average incomes reported by older men in 1901 were sufficient to support an aged couple, one must first know what the cost of living for two people in that year might have been. Unfortunately, there are few reliable contemporary sources from which to construct cost-of-living estimates.[19] The result has been that historians have been able to do little more than discern general trends in the relationship between prices and income. As David and Rosemary Gagan point out, "in spite of two decades of intensive research into the social history of late-Victorian Ontario, the standard of living associated with the growth of industrialization and urbanization is still an intriguing lacuna in our historical understanding."[20] The available information suggests, however, that the average income of $400 reported by aged men in 1901 was indeed sufficient to support an aged couple. Brian Gratton reports that in the United States expenditures for people over sixty amounted to $231 per person in 1891 and $319 per person in 1917. While both these estimates indicate that an aged couple spent more than $400 a year, Gratton notes that these expenditures included luxuries such as amusements, vacations, books, and newspapers. The aged, he discovered, were not living at subsistence level.[21]

In Canada, the Gagans calculated that an average working-class wage in 1889 was $450.[22] Gordon Darrach, however, suggests that manual labourers during the 1890s earned no more than $400 annually when they were fortunate enough to be fully employed, which was rare.[23] Terry Copp, meanwhile, remarks that a budget developed for the Child Welfare Exhibition in Montreal in 1912 determined that a family required at least $550 a year to meet subsistence level.[24] These amounts generally refer to the cost of maintaining a family of five. Few aged men were required to support this many dependants. Also, most cost-of-living calculations assume that a considerable portion of a family's income was spent on rent. The aged, however, were more likely than younger individuals to own their home, a fact that would reduce the amount they had to spend on shelter.[25] When one notes that in 1891 a family of five could subsist on $65 worth of food a year, and considering that inflation was minimal between 1891 and 1901,[26] it becomes obvious that an aged couple could, in all probability, survive quite easily on an income of $400 annually.

As well, Brian Gratton and Francis Rotundo argue that, rather than creating widespread poverty among the aged, industrialization engendered economic growth which had "very positive effects" for many aged people.[27] They note that aged people in the United States often survived on savings accumulated by combining the employment income of the entire family. When the income of adult children living at home was pooled, there was often not merely enough to meet living expenses but a surplus. Parents used this surplus to provide themselves with savings upon which they could rely during their retirement.

It is likely that many aged people in Ontario were able to supplement their employment income in this manner. In Brockville, Kingston, and St Catharines, large numbers of adult children lived in the homes of their aged parents. A majority of these children were employed. While it cannot be determined what portion of their income, if any, these individuals donated to their parents, Jane Synge's study suggests that the expectation was that children living at home would contribute the bulk of their earnings to their parents.[28] There is also evidence of older people accumulating assets during this period. David and Rosemary Gagan, for instance, remark that more people were saving more money in the latter decades of the century.[29]

In addition, Livio Di Matteo demonstrates that, among decedents in Wentworth County, older people held the largest share of real-estate wealth.[30] This would support Gratton's claim that the aged were more likely to receive non-employment income such as annuities from savings and rents. Michael Katz indicates, too, that elderly people often sold their homes to obtain money with which to live in their old age.[31] This would mean that the average employment income of $400 reported by Ontario's aged in 1901 was not necessarily their total income. It would also mean, as Gratton and Rotondo have suggested, that those people whose employment income was most certainly too low to support them, such as the 13 per cent of the aged men in St Catharines, Kingston, and Brockville who reported earnings of less than $200 a year, or those people who reported no employment income, may have nevertheless enjoyed a comfortable existence.

This hypothesis is supported by an examination of the wills of the aged people dying in Brockville between 1891 and 1915.[32] A total of eighty-three wills, thirty from women and fifty-three from men, representing 17 per cent of the aged population in the 1891 census, was located. These wills indicate that aged people in Ontario did indeed accumulate substantial assets aside from employment income on which they could live even when unemployed. Combined, the estates represented a total accumulation of wealth of over $650,600, an average of $7,830 for each estate. In reality, of course, this wealth was far from equally distributed among the population. The estates ranged from the $130 worth of property possessed by a widow named Margaret Quinn to the fortune of Samuel Flint, which was valued at $79,550. Most people, a total of 41 per cent of the decedents, left estates worth between $1,000 and $5,000. A further quarter of the estates were assessed at between $5,000 and $10,000. In all, 65 per cent of the estates fell into the medium category of $1,000 to $10,000. Wealthier people, those with estates of between $10,000 and $20,000, formed almost 10 per cent of the decedents, while the wealthiest segment of the estates, valued at over $20,000, comprised a further 10 per cent of the total. Relatively poor people, with estates valued at less than $999, made up 14 per cent of the total.

Half of the total wealth represented by these estates, a total of $320,550, was held in real estate. Almost three-quarters of the decedents possessed at least one town lot. Some held vast real-estate fortunes. Samuel Flint, for instance, held over $78,000 in buildings, lots, warehouses, and agricultural land.[33] William Sherwood, a lawyer, owned $25,000 in real estate.[34] Most people, over 60 per cent of those people holding such property, owned between $2,000 and $6,000 in real estate made up of one or two town lots and their residence.

Nearly one-quarter of the decedents possessed no real estate. Yet these individuals were not necessarily poor. While 37 per cent of the landless individuals had estates valued at less than $1,000, another 12 per cent possessed estates worth over $10,000. Edward Jolling, for instance, owned no real estate but left an estate worth $45,000.[35] Half of the landless individuals left estates of medium value, between $5,000 and $10,000.

The next most important category of wealth evident in the wills was savings or investment income, which represented 31 per cent of the total value of the estates. This type of wealth was distributed throughout a greater portion of the estates than was real estate. A total of 78 per cent of the decedents possessed savings, stocks, bonds, annuities, or life insurance. Most people merely put their savings in the bank, but over 17 per cent held stocks, bonds, or annuities while an equal number purchased life insurance. These investments, valued at a total of $205,291, represented a substantial amount of accumulated wealth and provided income in the form of interest payments or dividends on which the aged could survive. While half of the investment wealth was held by people with estates valued at over $10,000 (each person possessing an average of $9,250 in savings or investments), the bulk (two-thirds) of the people holding this type of wealth had medium-sized estates worth between $1,000 and $10,000. Each of these people held an average of $1,600 in savings or investments. Even the among poorest group of decedents, 60 per cent held some form of savings or investments, averaging $477 for each person. Though this was a relatively small amount of money, it is greater than the $400 reported as the average annual income of elderly people in Brockville in 1901.

A third indication of accumulated wealth and savings among the aged is the degree of wealth held in the form of loans and mortgages. The ability to loan money to others indicates that a person had excess income to distribute. Mortgages testify that a person once held real estate. They also represent a source of income. Over one-third of the inventories in the wills of Brockville's aged decedents listed monies secured by mortgages, promissory notes, or loans due. This finding supports Michael Katz's claim that aged people often sold their homes or property and lived off the proceeds.

Together, the information gathered from the wills of Brockville's aged citizens indicates that the situation in Ontario was similar to that described by Gratton and Rotondo for the United States. At least a portion of Brockville's aged population possessed substantial amounts of wealth. Even the poor segment of the population held property, savings, or investments which would permit them to survive without employment income. Certain wills suggest that this was the case. Sisters Margaret and Ester McGibbon, spinsters, were reported as living together in the 1891 census. Margaret died in 1897, leaving her entire estate, valued at $1,000, to Ester. Ester was seventy years old, unemployed, and with no visible income. While she may have had savings of her own, she presumably relied mainly upon her inheritance. When she died in 1900,

Ester left an estate of $450.[36] It appears that $1,000 was enough to support her for at least two years. Similarly, John Arnold, who possessed no real estate, left his wife, Abigail, an estate of $6,000 when he died in 1892. When she died four years later, her estate was valued at $4,250.[37] Although she may have had another source of income, it appears that Abigail could survive on less than $500 a year even though she presumably had to pay for her rent or lodgings.

The wills also refute the idea that all aged non-heads were dependent.[38] Sally Gates Booth and her husband David lived in the home of a friend. According to the census, they appear to have been an elderly couple without sufficient financial resources to maintain their own home. When Sally died in 1899 she left an estate of $62,300, one of the largest in Brockville.[39] Obviously, the Booths were not financially dependent and chose to live with friends for other reasons.

Evidence of the contributions of employed adult children living in the homes of their parents is offered by the case of Nellie Poulin. She and her husband appeared in the previous chapter as an example of an elderly couple living with several wage-earning adult children. One of these children, Peter, remained with his widowed mother, apparently contributing to her support until his death in 1907, when he left her an estate valued at over $11,000.[40] Obviously, despite having no source of income, Nellie Poulin lived comfortably while her son was alive and even after his death she possessed sufficient resources to permit her a comfortable existence.

The limited evidence offered here suggests that Gratton's hypothesis is correct and Ontario's aged did indeed manage to ward off dependency with more success than has been previously admitted. At the very least, we can conclude that reports of the widespread financial dependency of the aged during the latter part of the nineteenth century were most certainly exaggerated. The majority of these individuals lived independently and were employed. Of those aged people who worked, most earned enough to support themselves. In fact, some were able to accumulate savings and investments which they used to support themselves when they were no longer able to work. It also appears that children contributed to the support of their parents. This is not to argue that the aged were wealthy. While some, such as Sally Booth or Samuel Flint, obviously enjoyed luxuries, and others, like Ester McKibbons, were merely able to meet their basic needs, it seems that most lived as John and Abigail Arnold, somewhere in between. In any case, there is little evidence of widespread poverty or destitution.

There were a few people who had no savings, no employment income, or an income that was inadequate to provide for their needs. These people probably did suffer poverty and deprivation. However, such examples of poor old people should not be seen as proof of the connection between age and destitution. Instead, these people were most certainly merely experiencing a continuation of the poverty they had known in their earlier lives. In a period when the bulk of the working-class population lived at or just above the level of subsistence,[41] it should not be surprising that aged people suffered the same incidence of destitution as younger working-class men. Rather than proving that old age was itself a cause of poverty and destitution, this merely suggests that the aged were no more and no less financially secure than anyone else.

Dependency can be measured in ways other than financial. The ability of the aged to participate in their community and interact socially is also an indication of independence and self-sufficiency. As Carole Haber points out, it was widely believed in the latter decades of the last century that the aged, even those with ample financial resources, were mentally and physically unable to lead active or productive lives.[42] Across North America many advice manuals, books, articles, and published sermons described old age as a period of disengagement and decay. Thomas Cole reports that, from at least the middle of the nineteenth century, the dominant popular image of old age portrayed the period as "a dreary waste, unproductive and cheerless, characterized chiefly by rheumatism, imbecility and decay."[43]

Not all commentators promoted such an image. A minority of writers, such as Lydia Child and C.M. Kirkland, advocated an active, cheerful old age. They encouraged elderly women in particular to participate fully in life and to involve themselves in the activities and interests of the young.[44] For the most part, however, these writers were on the defensive. The dominant tendency to view the aged as worn out and unproductive persisted.

An investigation of the information available in newspapers, letters, diaries, and obituaries in Ontario suggests that the true circumstances of the aged may have been much closer to ideal promoted by writers such as Child and Kirkland than most historians have recognized. Admittedly, the bulk of the information provided here represents the wealthier portion of the aged population. This group tended to remain healthy and active longer than working-class individuals. It is also evident that people in clerical, professional, or non-manual occupations were able to pursue their careers longer than manual labourers, who were often forced by infirmity to give up their jobs. Nevertheless, examples of active, productive, and mentally capable older individuals of any class or income bracket certainly furnishes strong evidence that the association of age with dependency due to senility or mental decay was inaccurate.[45]

Ellen Osler (1806–1907) and Wilmot Cumberland (1811–93), for example, were two active elderly women who lived in Toronto during the late nineteenth century. Both were members of Toronto's privileged elite. Ellen was the wife of the Reverend Featherstone Lake Osler, one of Upper Canada's early missionary workers, and the mother of three of the most famous men in nineteenth-century Canada: the financier Edmund Osler, the surgeon William Osler, and Briton Bath Osler, the renowned lawyer. Wilmot, meanwhile was married to Frederick Cumberland (1821–81), the famous engineer, architect, and member of parliament. Both these women remained active, physically, mentally, and socially, well into old age. In fact, rather than being dependent in any way, both Ellen and Wilmot had others who required their care. Wilmot's husband, Frederick, was bedridden for months before his death, and throughout his illness she was his primary caregiver. Similarly, Ellen, even though she was in her eighties, spent several years caring for her invalid husband as he slowly deteriorated and died. Though both women had the advantage of large families and servants to assist them while caring for their husbands, they shouldered the emotional burden involved in such an endeavour and a great deal of the physical burden too. Yet they also found the time to lead active lives.

Ellen wrote to her son William in 1886, "The days slip by so quickly, there seems not time to do half I would like and you know the house is always busy."[46] She pointed out to her sister Lizzie, who was also elderly, that "I hear now and then of someone who has nothing to do and cannot tell how to manage and rid themselves of the time. That is not you, nor me either."[47] Even at eighty-three, Ellen had to plan her daily schedule to ensure that she accomplished all she wished, and she once remarked on the "steady stream of visitors [who] kept her distracted all day."[48] When she did feel unable to remain active all day long, she was quite frustrated and commented that she "could not understand feeling old."[49] It was not until she was over ninety, however, that she noted that "age and its many infirmities must excuse my many negligences."[50] As she approached her hundredth year Ellen fell ill and was bedridden. But she could still not stand to be confined. Unable to leave her room, she felt that "she was in prison."[51]

When over seventy, Wilmot Cumberland took care of her own finances, paid her own bills, and kept track of her budget and the amount of coal she used. She reported a hectic daily schedule which included French classes, charity works, attending meetings of the board for the Home for Incurables, attending the opera, and dancing until 2 a.m.[52] Even near the end of her life, Wilmot's schedule for one month included weekly meetings of the board for the Home for Incurables, a recital, a costume ball, "home business," and making pear preserves.[53]

She felt obliged to mention the days she remained at home and reported that "it was very dull and lazy of me."[54]

Ellen Osler and Wilmot Cumberland were not unique: their letters and diaries indicate that several of their aged friends and relatives were active and alert, and the same was true of many of their other contemporaries. The Reverend William Griffin (1827–1917) reported on his eightieth birthday that "after a man has reached the age of eighty he might reasonably be expected to retire, but I wish it distinctly understood that I am not of a retiring disposition."[55] Amelius Irving, the treasurer of the Law Society of Upper Canada, kept his position until he was almost ninety. Despite his age he seldom failed to put in an appearance at his office in Osgoode Hall every day it was open for business.[56] Meanwhile, upon his retirement at the age of eighty-four, George Cuddy of the Canada Trust Corporation stated that he felt "rather young to be quitting."[57] While documentation concerning the daily activities of people of humbler social station is not as abundant, there is enough to indicate that an active old age was not confined to the wealthier members of society. The Reverend William Cochrane, a rural minister who lived in constant fear of being unable to provide for his wife, reported visiting 325 families and travelling 11,920 miles the year he turned sixty-five.[58]

Two questions remain. If the bulk of the aged population was not financially, physically, or mentally dependent, why did the government encourage the public to believe that aged people were mainly ill, feeble-minded, and dependent upon public assistance? And why did the government blame families for this situation and insist that they were refusing to offer proper care to their aged relatives? The answer to both questions, it appears, is that popular images of old-age dependency and population aging were employed by the state to its own political advantage.

Several historians have discovered that the discrepancies between public perceptions of widespread dependency and crisis among the aged and the actual condition of the elderly population have usually been the result of political rhetoric. Jill Quadagno, for instance, argues that much of the emphasis on old-age poverty and dependency in the late nineteenth century was of political origin. She explains that information concerning the living situation of the aged was a "theme with political significance," used in different ways by opposing sides in debates over various social-welfare issues.[59] In the case of England, advocates of public pensions highlighted the plight of the destitute minority of the aged population in order to arouse public support for non-contributory pension legislation.[60] Government officials, meanwhile, used the rising incidence of institutionalization among the elderly as evidence of widespread lack of concern for the aged on the part of their families[61] and as justification for a reduction of public spending on the aged. Cutbacks in this area, it was claimed, would help to revive proper filial affections among the relatives of dependent older people.[62] As David Thomson notes, in England during the 1870s and 1880s, officials responsible for administering the Poor Law reduced the cost of outdoor relief by cutting off payments to aged people and forcing their families to support them instead.[63] While these measures were introduced mainly to save money, government officials explained that they were trying to recreate the sense of familial obligation between children and their parents which they insisted had been destroyed by the availability of overly generous public relief. "Only by cutting assistance to all," it was stated, "could the policy emphasizing self-responsibility be successful."[64] It appears that a similar sentiment guided the Ontario provincial government.

Similarly, Brian Gratton and Sue Weiller argue that the degree to which the elderly were being forced out of the American workforce prior to 1930 was exaggerated to create support for the implementation of social-security programs. Despite the stories of high levels of unemployment and dependency among the aged which were used to justify universal retirement policies, Gratton and Weiller explain that old-age pensions created rather than reflected major changes in the work and economic situation of the elderly. Instead of rescuing an unemployed and impoverished aged population from dependency, social security was initiated mainly to remove the aged from the labour force in order to open up jobs for unemployed younger men. The very fact that the aged had to be legislated out of the workforce suggests that their labour-force participation was considerable. In this sense, Weiller comments that the often-cited decrease in the labour-force participation of older men between 1890 and 1930 was more apparent than real and that the rhetoric around the issue was concerned more with political debates than with the real needs or condition of the aged themselves.[65]

In conclusion, many of assumptions that people hold concerning the dependency of the aged in the nineteenth century and the role that families played in their care are clearly inaccurate. Also, many of these false impressions were created or at least encouraged by government officials who manipulated public sentiment in order to justify policies of fiscal restraint. Families bore the brunt of the blame for what were often government-initiated policies based not on the needs of the aged but on political and financial considerations. The following chapters shall elaborate upon this process.

Families, Neighbours, and Communities: Local Support Systems for the Aged Poor in Nineteenth-Century Ontario

In the 1890s, much of the debate concerning the state's responsibilities towards the aged revolved around the issue of family obligations. This discussion rested upon two assumptions: that the care of the dependent aged had traditionally been the sole responsibility of their families, and that late-nineteenth-century families were shirking their responsibilities and refusing to provide the necessary care to their aged relatives. These assumptions became the basis of and justification for major policy decisions which redefined the boundaries between family obligations and state responsibilities and dramatically increased the degree to which families and, more particularly, younger generations were made responsible for the dependent aged. Considering the implications these policy changes had on the province's aged population and their families, it is important to understand that both of the assumptions underlying them were wrong. Prior to the 1890s, families were never expected to shoulder the entire burden of caring for the dependent aged. Furthermore, there is no evidence that nineteenth-century families became unwilling to provide care for their aged relatives.

An examination of municipal poor-relief records and a variety of sources such as diaries, letters, newspapers, and genealogies during the latter half of the nineteenth century reveals that, while families provided the bulk of the physical care required by their aged relatives, their local communities were willing to assist them with the task. Well before the advent of the modern welfare state, communal support networks that emphasized the social interdependence of individuals existed in most Ontario communities. These networks survived in one form or another until the final decades of the nineteenth century, when they began to decline because of provincial policy decisions. Under such a system, which caused Susannah Moodie to describe Upper Canadians as "a truly charitable people,"[1] the dependent aged were viewed as a community responsibility. When old people lacked the resources to support themselves, neighbours and friends usually ensured that they were provided for in their own homes or cared for by others in a way that did not disrupt their lives unnecessarily.[2]

Of course, providing charity to one's neighbours was not always an act of pure generosity. It was usually a combination of true benevolence and a strong sense of obligation that compelled people to help their neighbours. As Laurel Thatcher Ulrich explains, in eighteenth-century and nineteenth-century New England, women were expected to be good neighbours. Being a good neighbour involved obligations of charity, helpfulness, and sociability. Charity, in particular, was understood to include personal responsibility for the well-being of one's nearby neighbours.[3] As well, the concepts of individuality and self-reliance, as we understand them today, were unknown in these communities. To help any one member of the community was to help the entire community. In this way, providing food or clothing to a needy neighbour, even an unpopular one, was one way a person proved to be a useful member of the community. Ulrich also explains that this concept of "neighbourliness" was not confined to rural New England but was recognized in many other rural environments.[4]

The population of nineteenth-century Ontario certainly recognized a form of communal spirit and neighbourliness similar to that described by Ulrich. Rather than assuming that families were to shoulder the entire burden of caring for their dependent members, neighbours and even municipal councils and magistrates understood that there were limits to the amount of care and financial support a family member could be expected to offer. Consequently, neighbours and friends were willing to supplement the assistance provided for the aged by family members and, in the absence of kin, neighbours fed, clothed, and cared for old people who were too ill or feeble to provide for themselves. The aged, as part of this communal support network, were not only recipients of care. Aged people who were able to often supported and cared for other people in need.

While communal support networks understood that few families were able to provide for all the needs of their dependent members, families were still a vital source of support and care for the aged. Friends, neighbours, and public officials expected families to care for their aged relatives to the extent of their ability. When families had done all they could, however, the community, represented by neighbours and friends or, if necessary, the local government, was willing to offer assistance to needy aged people or their families.

Outside Ontario's few cities, the poor relief provided by municipal councils was usually the most important and often the only resource for the poor beyond the informal charity of friends.[5] Hence, while little is known about poor relief in mid-nineteenth-century Ontario,[6] petitions for relief received by local governments are the main source of information concerning how the destitute and infirm were cared for in this period. During most of the nineteenth century, people in Ontario could petition their local government councils for assistance when they were no longer able to provide for themselves. The petitions for aid received by the courts of the General Quarter Sessions of the Peace before 1850, and by the various municipal and county councils after that date, reveal much about families, communities, and the care of the dependent aged in nineteenth-century Ontario. Although these records are often incomplete and cover a broad range of communities over the course of several decades, one common feature of all the petitions is the testimony they offer of an overwhelming sense of community responsibility towards the dependant aged.

For present purposes, the term community shall be understood to encompass friends and neighbours as well as the local municipal, township, or county government bodies. As Lynne Marks indicates, the bulk of Ontario's nineteenth-century population experienced life in small towns; one-third of the province's population in 1891 resided in towns containing fewer than 5,000 people. Within these towns, the significance of personal ties and close social interaction blurred the divisions between the private, informal charity of friends and neighbours and the formal, public assistance offered by municipal councils and other local governments.[7] Where possible, the following discussion distinguishes between informal private charity and public charity. When the term community is used without qualification, however, it should be understood to include both.

English and American local governments had a variety of poor laws to guide their charitable actions, but Upper Canada, Canada West, and early Ontario did not. Although the Cataraqui memorial of 1768 stated that "humanity will not allow us to omit mentioning the necessity of appointing overseers of the poor, or the making of some kind of provision for persons of the description, who, from age or accident, may be rendered helpless,"[8] there was little official or legislative provision made in Upper Canada for the care of the indigent. This may have been because, in most cases, people in need could rely on the informal support of their community. Nevertheless, "from the earliest days of the history of Canada, the principle has been generally recognized that poor-relief may be granted legitimately from public funds."[9] Public relief, therefore, was seen as a legitimate and necessary extension of individual benevolence.[10] Also, as Mary Stokes has pointed out, the populace of mid-nineteenth-century Ontario trusted their local government to do what was "just" and "fair."[11] Hence, with or without formal guidelines or official recognition of formal public responsibility for the poor, individuals, families, or even entire communities felt justified, once their resources were exhausted, in seeking assistance from public funds by petitioning local officials.

Petitions outlined the supplicant's situation and gave reasons why the local officials should grant the aid. Generally, they assured officials that the individual in question had nowhere else to turn and that all other avenues of assistance had been exhausted. It was generally assumed that mutual support among neighbours had preceded and would accompany municipal relief.[12] There was nothing unusual about this. M.J. Heale explains that, in early-nineteenth-century New York State, individual and neighbourly action was a characteristic of rural benevolence. He argues that charity created a sense of community among settlers, binding them together by mutual ties and obligations.[13]

While David Murray has commented that Niagara District magistrates in the early nineteenth century were "niggardly" in granting relief to individuals,[14] it is likely that they were merely acting according to well-established traditions of poor relief; the assistance they provided to the poor was a supplement to communal relief, not a replacement.[15] This perspective included, it seems, the treatment of community support as a complement to family-based care rather than an alternative to it.[16] Following a tradition that had survived in England since medieval times, poor relief was regarded, in most instances, as merely one of several sources of support for the aged poor.[17] It was never the intention of the magistrates that people could live entirely on the relief they distributed.

This does not mean that the lives of the destitute elderly were pleasant or that they received all the care they needed. It must be remembered that the people who provided care for the aged were often poor themselves.[18] James Smith has calculated that few households had more than a minimal amount of disposable income to redistribute to needy neighbours and kin.[19] The charity of neighbours, therefore, however generous it may have been, was always "precarious and uncertain."[20] Nevertheless, the petitions reveal that communities did their best to provide care and financial assistance for those old people who were in need, regardless of whether they had living relatives or not.

As Jill Quadagno affirms, since so many poor survived despite the meagre amount of poor relief that was available, they were clearly supporting each other to a remarkable extent.[21] Communal support was also demonstrated by the fact that petitions were usually signed by several people who exhibited a concern for the individual in question by testifying that the applicant's statements were true and that he or she was indeed a worthy object of charity. Often these witnesses were friends and neighbours who had helped the applicant in the past and would, it was expected, continue to provide some assistance in the future. Another point to be kept in mind is that, in most of the townships and municipalities across the province, the councillors usually had personal knowledge of both the need and the circumstances of the various petitioners and their neighbours. This knowledge was frequently relied on in determining what amount of municipal relief would be just or fair in any given situation. In England, at least, E.W. Martin claims that the poor were usually well served by this system.[22]

In Upper Canada, before 1850, the magistrates of the courts of Quarter Sessions in each district were actually given no authority by legislation to provide aid to for the destitute.[23] The population in general, however, supported the extension of relief to the indigent. Consequently, grand juries encouraged magistrates to "deliver such as are really in distress by making proper provisions for the same."[24] Among magistrates as well, Allan Irving reports, there existed "the willingness ultimately to expend public funds."[25] As a result, courts frequently played an ad hoc role in assisting the destitute by voting expenditures to meet the needs of those people they deemed most worthy of support.[26] Similar to the situation David Thomson found in England, pleas for assistance from the aged or requests made on behalf of old people met with a favourable response in Upper Canada's courts.[27]

The lack of legislative authority in these matters, however, allowed some districts to refuse aid without having to explain why. The magistrates of the Niagara District, for instance, frequently rejected applications for aid on the grounds that "no funds are provided by law."[28] David Murray claims that the apparent unwillingness of the magistrates to help the poor after 1829 was due to cold heartedness[29]; however, their attitude almost certainly had more to do with the depleted state of the district treasury than with any personal callousness. It also seems that, although the general public in Niagara frequently objected to the magistrates' refusal to support the poor, they did understand that the cost of such activities was a significant issue. For example, when the question of erecting a public residence for the poor arose, the grand jury responded to the magistrates' unwillingness to spend any funds on such a project by announcing that "if the expense be a matter of consideration to council the citizens generally would sustain any action in the matter."[30]

Despite the apparent willingness of the populace to accept a degree of public responsibility for the care of the poor, official legislation regarding local poor relief was slow to develop. During the 1830s various municipalities were granted the right to distribute poor relief in their charters. In 1849, the Municipal Incorporation Act officially granted responsibility for supporting the poor to newly formed county councils. In many cases, however, the act restricted poor relief, since it placed in question municipalities' rights to perform the relief activities they had formerly carried out on an informal basis. The formal power to grant outdoor relief, or monetary aid, was officially extended to town councils only a decade later. Originally, municipalities required the assent of the majority of the ratepayers to levy a special tax to raise money for the support of the poor. By 1866, however, municipalities were allowed to appropriate funds for poor relief from the general revenue. People seeking aid would petition these councils in the same manner in which they had previously sought aid from the district courts. Still, the legislation that brought about these changes left the provision of aid by municipalities permissive rather than obligatory.[31]

The informal nature of most communal support systems makes the subject difficult to study. Petitions are among the few documents that provide any details concerning how communities cared for the aged, however, even the aid granted by local magistrates and municipal councils was often deemed to be peripheral to the activities of the municipality and hence few councils kept complete or detailed records of their responses to the various poor-relief petitions they received. Nevertheless, although only a few petitions exist for any one region or period, once these scattered clusters of petitions from the several municipalities and districts of the province are combined, a large body of information emerges.[32]

Unfortunately, it is often difficult to determine whether these petitions were granted or rejected. It is also not possible to ascertain if the relief granted was adequate. Because of these problems, a detailed analysis of how local officials responded to people's pleas for help is not possible, nor is any form of statistical analysis. That said, the petitions remain a valuable source of information; for, regardless of whether the petitioners' requests were accepted or rejected, or whether the aid granted was sufficient or not, the information in the petitions themselves reveals much about community support networks and the role they played in the lives of the dependent aged in nineteenth-century Ontario.

As already indicated, the petitions make clear that, at both the informal and the formal level, society accepted a large degree of responsibility for supporting the aged and the people who cared for them. There was a general conviction that the community as a whole had a special responsibility to assist those elderly people who had served it in one way or another. Individuals and communities alike believed that serving as a local official, fighting in the army, or having provided care for others in need all qualified a person as especially worthy of financial support.

On several occasions communities petitioned local municipal councils on behalf of elderly people they felt were deserving of assistance. The people of East Gwillimbury, for instance, felt that Thomas Kelly had "strong claims upon his countrymen" since he had been a soldier for twenty-eight years and had fought with the Duke of Wellington in the Peninsular Wars.[33] Similarly, Isabella Lee of Burford Township was recommended for aid in 1850 because she was the widow of a British soldier.[34] Likewise, Elizabeth James, who at the age of eighty became feeble and almost helpless, was found to be a proper object of public charity because she had two adult daughters, one blind, the other insane, whom she had done "her utmost to support ... while she was able."[35]

Being a long-time member of the community also qualified people for aid. It was felt that early settlers who had experienced "the toils and privations peculiar to new and remote settlements"[36] helped develop communities to the benefit of those people who arrived later and so were deserving of community support. For example, twenty-eight residents of Raleigh Township petitioned the municipal council to provide aid for Mary Berkley, an elderly indigent widow, because she had been in the community "since the early days of settlement."[37] The people of the same township also regarded it as their "duty" to approach council on behalf of a Mr James, who was unable to work owing to rheumatism and other ailments associated with old age, because he was "one of our life long residents."[38]

Despite the willingness of communities to seek municipal aid on behalf of aged individuals, the most common theme among the petitions from aged people themselves is that they had no desire to request public assistance. Older people, it seems, were determined to remain independent as long as possible. Most considered petitioning the local council for aid only as a desperate last resort once all other avenues of support had been exhausted. And even then, it was the "infirmities which accompany age" and not age in itself that usually prompted them to apply for help. The petitions reveal that people did not think that they were deserving of public support, regardless of how old they were, as long as they were healthy enough to work and earn a living for themselves. For example, eighty-year-old Thomas Thrush stated that he had been determined to provide for himself as long as he could. He recalled that he had been "for these many years tossed about from one place to another to obtain the small pittance which helped to sustain me." Only once he found himself too feeble to continue this type of life did he petition the Niagara town council for assistance. Even then he "found himself reluctant to sit down in [his] situation of want and necessity," but he hoped "some kind friend ... would sympathize for [him]."[39] Similarly, Mrs Gordon assured the members of the Pittsburgh Township council that necessity brought about by age and its accompaniments, weakness and infirmity, and not "any irregularity or extravagances" on her part, had left her dependent on the charity of council. She added that, if her health would permit her to gain a maintenance, "she indeed would shrink from the idea of adding to their already onerous duties."[40]

Even once they were too ill or too weak to work, few aged people applied for public aid until they had made every effort to find alternative means of support. For instance, in 1823 Spraig Frusley explained that after thirty years in the Newcastle District he found himself with no choice but to request aid from the magistrates: "quite unable to do the last thing for a living" because of old age and infirmities, he was also without home or property of any kind and lacked any friends able to maintain and keep him.[41] Like Spraig, most petitioners asked for relief only once they realized that they could not survive without it. Stephen Smith of Elizabethtown, for example, found himself in this situation. He had been crippled in an accident when he was fifty-six and could not work. Nevertheless, he managed to provide for himself, by one means or another, for a full ten years. By that point, however, "he had exhausted all the means he ever had to support himself" and was forced to request aid from the Leeds and Grenville county council.[42]

When they did apply for assistance, most aged people felt they had strong claims on community funds. Few claimed that age or infirmity alone entitled them to support; instead, most appealed to principles of communal reciprocity and interdependence among neighbours.[43] They felt that just as the time they had spent raising their family entitled them to support from their children, the contributions they had made to their community during their lifetime justified their request for communal support. John Moore of the Niagara District, for example, recounted the story of his life to the magistrates of the court of the General Quarter Sessions. In his petition of 1832 he explained that he had been a soldier in Portugal, a settler in New York State, and finally a Loyalist refugee in the Niagara region. He had acted as a township assessor for thirteen years and taught school throughout the Niagara District. He had also served as a school trustee and in that capacity was responsible for encouraging the central government of the colony to fund schools in the region. Even once he was over the age of seventy, he continued to teach at several schools to earn his livelihood, a routine that entailed considerable travel. Unfortunately, he discovered that the pay he received was too low to permit him to save for his future sustenance. Hence, he found himself, "at the advanced age of ninety years, helpless, infirm [and] destitute of the means of existence." He hoped that the years of service that he rendered to the inhabitants of the district would be deemed sufficient to warrant granting him a small pension "to preserve him during the brief remainder of his days."[44]

Similarly, Elizabeth Thomson was left "in strained circumstances" when her husband, a member of parliament, died while attending the legislature. She believed that her husband's services to his community should entitle her to aid.[45] Edward Walker also felt himself deserving of assistance considering that he was wounded three times while fighting in the War of 1812. He hoped that in return "for all his services and wounds" he would be "granted a pension in his old age."[46] Likewise, Henry Hayes petitioned the county council of Leeds and Grenville in 1871. The independent ninety-year-old found himself "wanting of money" but did not wish the councilmen to provide him charity. He only wanted to secure the support he felt he was entitled to because of the services he had performed for his countrymen as a soldier in 1837. He had failed to obtain the proper paper work when he left the army, however, and so he could not claim his pension. He also knew that tracking down the necessary records would require more money than he had available. Thus, he merely asked the council to help defray the expenses he would incur in trying to obtain his pension. Once acquired, he argued, the pension would allow him to support himself for the rest of his life, independent of the council's support.[47]

Communities did not limit their generosity to only those old people who could prove they had contributed to the community in some manner. Friends and neighbours often petitioned their local councils for aid simply because an elderly person was in need and they felt unable to provide for that individual without formal municipal assistance. For instance, the neighbours of Charlotte Coogan were genuinely concerned for her well-being and wished to provide care for her. Unfortunately, they were unable to do so on their own. For this reason, they petitioned the Leeds and Grenville county council for assistance. Noting that Charlotte suffered from mental infirmity as well as the bodily infirmities of age and would often fall in the highway, "exposing herself to the danger of a sudden and unprovided for death," the petitioners "craved a small donation from the council to enable them to provide for her some safe abode."[48] In another instance, twenty-three people petitioned their municipal council for aid to Christopher Gallagher and his wife, who were both over seventy years old, destitute, and "dependent upon the kindness of their neighbours." The entire neighbourhood, it was noted, "has for a long time rendered ... such relief as thought best." Having done what it could the community hoped that the council would now take over the responsibility of supporting the aged couple.[49] Likewise, Larkin Parish, aged eighty-seven, "an old worn out soldier ... destitute of any support," was cared for by "the charitable and humane part of the community" until they found the burden too onerous and requested assistance from the local magistrates.[50] In another example, the inhabitants of East Gwillimbury suggested that the council levy a special tax upon all the ratepayers in order to raise money to help Michael Carle, an old infirm man who was unable to support himself.[51]

While local communities accepted the principle that they had a certain responsibility to support the aged poor, local officials were not willing to do so unless it was absolutely necessary. Regardless of how deserving someone may have been, communities expected each member of the community, the aged included, to tend to their own individual needs to the best of their ability. Those people who could not provide for themselves were expected to turn to their relatives before they requested either formal or informal communal support.

Community values, then, did include the notion that families should provide a certain degree of care for their dependent kin. And it appears that most families did what the community expected. Prior to the 1890s there is little indication in public records, such as petitions for aid, that families were failing to furnish what the community deemed to be sufficient amounts of care for their aged relatives. Though it is difficult to determine exactly what type of care or what quantity of care families provided, it is clear that caring for dependent family members, especially an aged relative, was fairly common. In fact, it was so common that few people thought it necessary to record their caregiving activities. Usually, family caregiving was discussed only when a problem arose.

As a result, the existing petitions are biased towards the more problematic instances of family care, ones where the family was forced to seek assistance or where families were found to be providing inadequate care, in most cases, families caring for an aged person never arrived at the point where they had to apply for municipal assistance. Thus, while petitions provide useful glimpses of caregiving activities and the various roles of the family, the community, and the local government in this process, the picture they present is incomplete. To obtain a fuller sense of the role of the family in providing care for the aged, it is necessary to supplement the information in the petitions with that found in a variety of other contemporary sources such as diaries, letters, and census records.

Historians such as Michael Anderson have suggested that nineteenth-century families usually assisted only those old people who could reciprocate in some way or those whose dependency was short term. People who possessed few resources or whose dependency was likely to be prolonged, it is supposed, were in danger of being ejected from or abandoned by the family.[52] Jill Quadagno refutes these claims. In her study of the Ribbon Weavers of Chilvers Cotton, England, between 1851 and 1901, she determined that families did their best to care for the aged even when there was little possibility of them providing any form of reciprocal service. She argues that the instances of institutionalization she did locate were acts of necessity due to economic hardship and cannot be interpreted as evidence of any desire on the part of nineteenth-century families to abandon the aged.[53]

Nevertheless, while numerous studies have dismissed as myth the notion that older people were frequently abandoned or neglected by their families,[54] it remains clear that several complex factors played a role in determining whether or not a relative felt able to provide care for an aged person. Today, most children accept that they should provide emotional, financial, and physical support for their elderly parents; however, some children do not feel capable of doing all they would like to.[55] This problem is hardly new. Anne McDonnell, a relatively wealthy Upper Canadian of United Empire Loyalist descent, discovered this same dilemma in 1805 when she returned to New York State to visit her aging parents who needed care. Her diaries indicate that she loved her parents dearly and was well aware of the "duty incumbent on a child to parents in the decline of life." Yet, though she often asked herself, "how can I pain them by soon leaving them," she decided that "I must go." When faced with the difficult choice of remaining to care for her parents or returning to her husband, Anne found that "the authority, the love of a husband even out does that of a parent." On her way home to her husband, Anne concluded that "if I did wrong to leave my parents, it is now too late to remedy it."[56]

Anne McDonnell's diary illustrates well the conflicts that could arise between the various responsibilities individuals had to their parents, their spouse, their children, and to other kin, as well as to themselves and their communities. As Emily Abel reports, caregiving for the ill or disabled aged was usually a function performed by wives or daughters. Aside from the well-meaning but rarely sufficient help of neighbours and other kin, these women often had to shoulder the entire burden of what could amount to around-the-clock care for their aged kin. Few of these caregivers had any professional training or medical knowledge, and only rarely did they have sufficient access to people who did.[57] Even if the elderly concerned required no specialized care, family members were at the very least obligated to bathe them, wash their clothes and sheets, cook special foods for them, and prepare their medications.

When these extra tasks were combined with the normal work of caring for a family and running a nineteenth-century household, it is easy to understand how the workload could become unbearable.[58] This was especially true if an aged person became senile and began to wander, act aggressively, or exhibit inappropriate sexual behaviour.[59] Frequently, when an illness progressed to this stage, the families and individuals who were providing care could simply not cope.[60]

The decision to care for an elderly person in need of assistance required taking all of these factors into consideration. In certain circumstances, one or more of them forced a person or even an entire family to decide that they could not provide the necessary care. Nevertheless, it appears that families who ended their caregiving functions were always the exception. This was the conclusion that Brian Gratton reached in his investigation of dependent aged people in Boston between 1890 and 1930. Even though economic and demographic considerations created a situation in which conflicting responsibilities and financial difficulties made it increasingly difficult for children to care for their aged parents, the portion of aged population found living with their children changed little. Rather than witnessing a decline in the degree to which families cared for the aged, the period after 1890 saw adult offspring and other kin working harder to maintain the dependent elderly.[61] Gratton concludes that, for every person forced to ask for public assistance, many more relied on adult children or other relatives for their food, lodging, and nursing care.[62]

Similarly, in Ontario there is no evidence that families became less willing to provide care as the century progressed despite the fact that it was increasingly difficult for them to do so. As Janet Finch explains, there have been variations and fluctuations in both people's need for support and the capacity of their kin to provide it. Moreover, demographic changes have meant that there have been periodic fluctuations in the existence of kin able to offer support.[63] Such was the case in nineteenth-century Ontario. The number of aged people in need of care was growing while families were becoming smaller.[64] As well, people experienced greater geographic mobility. As one newspaper commented, "keeping up the family attachment" was difficult when business and other pursuits scattered family members to distant homes.[65] One result of these trends was that by the time parents reached old age they often found that there were fewer people nearby to provide them with care.[66] Another, as Ann Orloff explains, was that "the proportion of adults at risk of supporting an elderly relative increased."[67] Increased mobility also meant that kin and communal support networks, which had often been a source of support for caregivers, were weakened.[68] Nevertheless, throughout the latter half of the nineteenth century, the degree to which Ontario's families sheltered their dependent elders remained unchanged.[69]

As the census schedules for Brockville, Kingston, and St Catharines reveal, throughout the latter half of the nineteenth century, children and other kin played a significant role in assisting the aged. While the mere fact of living with a child or relative does not prove that the aged were cared for, contemporary studies affirm that if aged parents require assistance their children usually provide it.[70] It is difficult to ascertain exactly what occurred within nineteenth-century homes, but what evidence there is suggests that they, too, provided care when it was needed.

William George Waind's reminiscences about his childhood in rural Ontario, for instance, contain several references to aged people being cared for by kin. One of them was his own grandfather: "My grandmother died and then my grandfather was left. He had a little money but not very much. The family had to keep him. There were five of them and they all had their turn."[71] A neighbour, Waind reported, built his mother a log house between his own home and his barn. "He thought it was a good place to have her, because he could visit her on his way to the barn and back."[72]

The genealogy of the Crawford family, which extends from the middle of the nineteenth century to the early part of the twentieth, offers further indication of the degree to which Ontario families supported the aged. Benjamin Crawford had thirteen children. He died while living with one of them. Of the other children who lived to old age, five were living with their spouse when they died and six others died in the homes of their children or their siblings.[73] Obituaries for aged people found in local newspapers often record that the deceased lived with kin. In one family, two sisters aged ninety-nine and ninety-four each lived with their sons. Another woman aged 101 had spent thirty-three years with her son.[74]

Ellen Osler's letters, written between 1870 and 1900, frequently refer to family members caring for elderly kin. She often lamented that her niece, Hattie, could never visit her. Every time Ellen invited her, Hattie replied that she felt "that she could not leave her mother just now, for she still requires attendance and much nourishment in the night."[75] Ellen's letters also reveal the extent to which family members who did not reside with the aged assisted them and their caregivers. During the years she spent caring for her husband, Ellen's son William, who lived in Baltimore, sent her advice and instructions on how to cope with her husband's deteriorating condition. As well, Ellen was frequently assisted in her caregiving activities by her daughters-in-law, grandnieces, and nieces, who would take turns spending a few days with her. In the final years of her life, Ellen herself received care from these same people. Similarly, Wilmot Cumberland's sister commented that should Wilmot require assistance her daughters "would consider it their first duty to attend to your wants." In addition, she noted that Wilmot was blessed "in having such a good son and wife so ready to show you affection."[76]

Not all aged people in need received help from their families. Those, for example, who required not lodging or nursing care but financial support often had to turn elsewhere. In England and United States, this fact was recognized by local communities. Janet Finch explains that in communities and families alike there was no automatic assumption of financial responsibility for elderly parents.[77] Instead, neighbours and municipal officials were willing to assist the aged with donations of food, fuel, or financial support. Historians such as Peter Laslett have confirmed that in the majority of cases financial contributions received from what he calls the collectivity, which included the local government as well as friends and neighbours, were far more vital to the aged than similar support offered by family members.[78] Although families provided most of the care needed by their aged kin, when a family could no longer shoulder the financial burden of caring for an aged relative, the community helped provide the assistance that person needed.[79] In this sense, community support networks played a vital role in the care of the aged. The mid-nineteenth-century definition of family obligations, therefore, was fluid and took individual circumstances into consideration. Communities recognized the limitations of family care and accepted responsibility for assisting not only the aged but also the people who cared for them.

Studies of poor-relief practices across North America confirm this statement. Robert Cray found that, during the eighteenth century and most of the nineteenth, local communities in the United States attempted as best they could to assist their destitute neighbours, balancing compassion with economy and benevolence with discipline. Often, he asserts, the care of the poor involved a large segment of the community.[80] Similarly, Virginia Burnhard discovered that American parishes in this period shared the responsibility for the aged poor, providing food, clothing, and shelter in a manner "characterized by generosity and neighbourly warmth."[81] It was also common for local authorities to issue small pensions, often referred to as "outdoor relief," to older people in need of assistance. As Priscilla Clement explains, this form of assistance was particularly useful since outdoor pensions were a humane way of dealing with poverty. They permitted the poor to remain in their community, in their own homes, and helped the aged by providing them with nursing care or shelter and by covering the cost of food or medicines.[82]

Like sentiments guided Ontarians. The population of Upper Canada felt that it was their "duty as christians to join hearts and hands to furnish the means of subsistence to our fellow beings"[83] and that "we should even incommode ourselves not a little" to aid a poor neighbour.[84] It seems that most people reacted as Alice Patterson did when she heard of a poor girl in her neighbourhood: "the conviction that I should do something for her forced itself upon me."[85] As well, Mary Gapper O'Brien recorded how her neighbours believed that they must "sacrifice" for "the benefit of others."[86] Together, they formed a communal support network which cared for those people who found themselves unable to provide for themselves. Several members of her community supported a man with "no visible means of support but the good offices of his friends."[87] Similarly, a poor Irish immigrant "lived on his neighbours," who had the "satisfaction of learning that [their] charity had not been misapplied," and[88] an indigent old man and his idiot daughter owed the cottage they lived in and the land they farmed "to the benevolence of a friend."[89]

Communities exhibited a particular concern for the aged. Although families were expected to provided what care they could, there is little evidence either of communities forcing kin to care for the aged or of people with relatives being excluded from receiving assistance. In a situation similar to that of England prior to 1880, it was a general policy to allow small amounts of out relief to the aged "without specific concern about pressuring children to contribute."[90] Usually, as was case with a poor widow who was supported wholly by the "charity of those know her" because her relatives could not render her any assistance in a "pecuniary way,"[91] communities felt obliged to provide assistance for individuals when family members could not.

Communities were aware that few individuals possessed the resources necessary to provide for all the needs of a dependent aged person. While one particular relative or neighbour might assume the bulk of the responsibility for any one such person, the rest of the community usually assisted them. When the entire community finally felt unable to provide sufficient aid, they often applied as a group for support from their local municipal or county councils, or they lent their support to the application of an aged person to ensure that that individual received the care he or she needed.

Although most aged people in need of care would turn to their families, those who had no kin could appeal only to the kindness of their neighbours. The petitions reveal that neighbours frequently took into their homes aged people who were simply too feeble or ill to live on their own or who had no means of providing themselves with shelter. Many of these people were eventually forced to request public assistance to help defray the added costs of feeding and sheltering an extra person; however, they usually did so only after they had been providing care for a considerable length of time. George Docstatder of Haldimand, for instance, cared for Henry Hard, a destitute, blind, and deaf eighty-seven-year-old man, for over a year before he asked for his municipal council to help him pay for Hard's maintenance.[92]

Neighbours often assumed the care of individuals who were already being cared for by kin but who were left alone because of the death or illness of their caregiver. This was the case with widow Cushing of Pittsburgh Township. She was cared for by her son until 1859, when he was killed in an accident while performing his statute labour for the township. Since he was the woman's only source of support, she was left dependent upon the charity of her neighbours. As a group, these neighbours petitioned the municipal council and obtained a grant for her support.[93] Similarly, when John Evans of Niagara was drowned, his neighbours urged the magistrates to provide some form of support for his widow, Eleanor, a woman of "upwards of seventy years of age" who was now alone and destitute.[94]

In other cases, communities took over the care of an aged person because it was obvious that their family was not caring for them adequately. Such was the case with Elizabeth Bowens. Her neighbours brought her appalling story to the attention of the magistrates of the Northumberland District Quarter Sessions in 1833. As a young woman, Bowens had been blinded and disfigured by smallpox and then abandoned by her husband. She found a home with her father for several years until he died. Afterwards, she was forced to turn to her brother for help. The aged woman signed over all her property to him; in return, he promised to feed, shelter, and care for her. The care he provided for Elizabeth consisted of confining her in a small unheated room and allowing no one to visit her. The blind old woman was forced to crawl over the ground in search of sticks and cow-chips to use as fuel to heat her room. Elizabeth finally managed to escape from her prison by feeling her way along fences until she found someone to help her.[95] Her neighbours hoped that the magistrates would offer Elizabeth a weekly provision for her support so that she could be cared by the community rather than by her brother.

Not only did people care for their relatives, friends, and neighbours, they also were frequently surprisingly generous to complete strangers. Doctor McLeod of East Gwillimbury attended upon a aged female vagrant for over three weeks before she died in his home; he had provided her with medical care and hired an assistant to look after her.[96]

Similarly, Alexander Ouellette of Essex County cared for, fed, and clothed an ill indigent man for over three months.[97] Tragically, an old man by the name of Surby took in a stranger who was afflicted with cholera. Surby generously provided what care he could for the man, only to die of the disease himself.[98]

As the case of Surby shows, the elderly were not always the recipients of care. They were also often caregivers for other dependent people. Widow Gibson had two orphaned and crippled grandchildren to care for. She realized that, if her grandchildren were ever to provide for themselves, they had to be educated. Claiming that, "though deformed in their limbs, [they] are blessed with good mental capacity and a great desire for learning," she attempted to educate them herself; however she found that, as she aged, she was not able to continue. Since she knew that she was near the end of her life, she urged the magistrates of her district to help the children obtain the education she could no longer provide for them.[99] Equally devoted to caring for a helpless relative, Samuel Enslow, a man greatly advanced in years, devoted his life to caring for his insane son. The latter required such constant care that Enslow was unable to earn a living to support his family. In 1849 his neighbours petitioned the district council for aid on his behalf.[100] Eleven years later a census enumerator visited Enslow and found him still caring for this son, who was by then so uncontrollable that he had to be tied down. The old man, it was reported, was "going down physically by the loss of his rest." Enslow's wife, however, refused to allow the son to be sent to an asylum. The enumerator suggested that the municipal council pay for someone to help Enslow care for the deranged offspring.[101]

In many cases, the aged also provided care for people who were not relatives. Pheobe Goodall, herself a widow "considerably advanced in life and of infirm health," took in an insane girl and cared for her, "consequently (exposing) herself and her family to the greatest privation."[102] One old man, Michael Kenny of Kitley Township, "through compassion and kind feeling" took in Margaret Hunter, a poor blind widow with no home, no money, and no friends." Kenny's neighbours, however, noted that he and his wife were in "declining life" and were really unable to care for Hunter. Consequently, they requested that the county council remunerate Kenney for the care he had provided and remove Hunter to another location both for her good and for Kenny's.[103]

Sometimes relatives applied for financial assistance when they found themselves overwhelmed by the burden of providing care. Thomas Angleman, for instance, was unable to support all his dependent relatives. His parents were "old and feeble and dependent upon him for their maintenance." This couple had also been caring for an orphaned "idiot" grandson until they were no longer able to do so. While Thomas was "willing to support his parents to the utmost of his ability," he explained that he was simply not able to "bear the burden of all three, having a family of his own to support." Hence, while he sought no help for his parents, in 1835 he requested that the magistrates of the Niagara District provide a weekly allowance for his nephew's support.[104] His request was granted.

Often, however, people caring for an elderly relative or neighbour never did request remuneration; instead, the elderly individuals or the community as a whole often requested that their local councils recognize the efforts of these kind people. Joseph Palmer, for instance, petitioned the county council of Leeds and Grenville on behalf of Mrs Stevens, the woman who had taken him in and cared for him. As he explained, "but for the charity and kindness and attentions of Mrs. Stevens, I must have perished from want."[105] Likewise, William Armstrong of Niagara, "infirm in body and almost blind and being destitute of friends and home," found himself, at the age of eighty-three, "under necessity of seeking a place among the humane and benevolent." He was eventually taken into the home of Daniel Burrowes, where he was provided with shelter and care for over six years. In 1849 Armstrong requested that he be provided with some money with which he could repay Burrowes for his kindness.[106] Meanwhile, the Niagara neighbours of John Burns and his wife felt that the couple deserved some financial aid in return for the trouble they experienced in taking care of an old and helpless woman.[107]

CONCLUSION

It is frequently mentioned that the level of care people received from their neighbours was minimal. Admittedly, there was a definite limit to both the quantity and the quality of the care any of these people could provide. Yet it must be reiterated that most of the caregivers mentioned in petitions were themselves poor; no matter how much they may have desired to provide sufficient care for a needy old person, their ability to do so was usually severely limited. Care in most of these instances consisted of furnishing the barest of necessities required to keep a destitute aged person alive. The information in the petitions suggests that, although communities may have been willing to do their utmost for the dependent and the destitute, communal care was rarely more than barely adequate. This, however, does not alter the fact that to a large extent neighbours and friends devoted what amounted to a large portion of their own meagre resources towards helping others. Despite the minimal amount of care they were able to supply, the generosity and kindness evidenced in the petitions should not be understated.

This generosity extended to aged people with families as well as to those without. The petitions reveal that families did not have to provide for all the needs of their aged members with no support or assistance from the community. While families may have been expected to shoulder the major portion of the burden of caring for the ill or dependent aged, neighbours and friends were willing to assist with the task. The petitions also reveal that communities felt that families struggling to care for dependent members were deserving of assistance from public funds. It was this sentiment of community support for the aged and for those who were caring for them that allowed many elderly to remain in their own homes or in the homes of their caregivers.

By the 1890s, however, the situation was changing. Gradually, throughout the final decades of the nineteenth century, responsibility for social welfare had been removed from the local municipal sphere and placed in the hands of provincial government authorities. As the province gained control over poor-relief practices, policies were initiated that placed a steadily increasing level of responsibility upon families. Government officials became unwilling to provide assistance to aged people with relatives and they refused to acknowledge that families caring for aged kin required support. Instead, they demanded that families do more for their aged kin. The fact that families were regularly unable to meet these new demands is evidenced by the frequent complaints of government officials concerning "irresponsible families." 🖋

Despite these complaints, families were no less willing to care for the aged at the end of the century than they had been earlier. What changed was not the amount of care families actually provided for the aged but the amount of care they were *expected* to provide. As the next chapter shall elaborate, provincial policies that accepted a decreasing degree of public responsibility for the aged poor helped change concepts of familial obligations towards the aged. These same policies also worked to undermine and even destroy communal support networks. The result was that, by the end of the nineteenth century, families caring for the aged were forced to shoulder the entire burden of care with little hope of formal assistance from either the state or their local communities.

Was gov't really formed

Government Policy towards the Dependent Aged in Ontario: Institutions and the Ideal Family

Just as the state has enacted major changes in the social-welfare system during the last fifty years, the second half of the nineteenth century also witnessed a significant transformation in poor-relief policies. Similar to recent policy changes related to the aged, the "great transformation of social experience," as Michael Katz describes it,[1] and the alterations in social policy that accompanied it during the middle and latter decades of the nineteenth century had an important impact on the lives of the indigent aged in Ontario.

During the later half of the nineteenth century, the Ontario government came to accept a great deal of responsibility for the care of the dependent aged. Its attention was, to a large degree, focused upon its own role in providing institutional forms of care. By the 1890s, however, panic over the increasing burden these responsibilities represented to the state treasury led provincial policy makers to re-evaluate their commitments to the aged. In particular, policy makers became concerned with reducing the number of aged people housed in institutions. This re-evaluation was guided by predictions of massive increases in the size of the aged population and the costs associated with caring for them.

In enacting such policies the Ontario government was hardly alone; governments in the United States and Great Britain also attempted to reduce social-welfare spending by forcing families to accept a larger share of responsibility for the care of the dependent elderly, especially their financial support. Their efforts in this regard were prompted, not by a decline in family responsibility towards the aged, but by their own fiscal priorities.

Priscilla Clement asserts that three motives guided welfare policies in the nineteenth century; genuine concern, social control, and fiscal restraint. All three affected policy, and none was ever totally absent, but the relative importance of each varied considerably over time.[2] David

Thomson adds that, regarding the support of the aged in particular, there has been a series of shifts between two loci of responsibility, namely the family and the community. The balance of responsibilities between these two poles has changed through the years in response to a multitude of social, economic, demographic, and political pressures.[3] When genuine concern was the primary motive of poor-relief policies, the balance of responsibility for the aged rested with the community; when fiscal restraint was the dominant consideration, policies were enacted to shift the bulk of the responsibility onto the family.

Historical research indicates that, traditionally, welfare policies in England and the United States emphasized the responsibility of the community to assist the aged and their families. David Thomson and others have located evidence that poor relief for the aged was "largely benevolent and sympathetic in operation."[4] While some historians have questioned Thomson's claims,[5] he asserts that nineteenth-century outdoor pensions for the aged were fairly generous, amounting to as much as between 70 and 80 per cent of the average working-class wage. Public pensions today, he points out, rarely provide the aged with more than 40 per cent of the average adult income.[6] Also, despite a lack of legal obligation, and in contradiction to the assumption that public pensions for the aged are a recent invention, Richard Smith asserts that most English communities made these pensions widely available to the aged. In doing so, he notes, society acted on the commonly accepted assumption that the elderly had a valid claim upon their community for support.[7] David Thomson contends that during this period a majority of the elderly working class received regular out door relief payments under the Poor Law. In fact, he calculates, between 65 and 70 per cent of all women over the age of seventy received some form of pension.[8]

Various historians have also discovered that poor-relief payments were not made only when the aged had no family nearby. Although it is often assumed that the presence of kin automatically rendered a person ineligible for public assistance, historians such as Jill Quadagno, David Thomson, and Richard Smith have pointed out that for the bulk of the nineteenth century poor-relief payments were distributed among the aged whether they had relatives or not and little attempt was made to recoup any part of this expenditure from the relatives who were legally liable to contribute. Even children, they argue, were almost never forced to help support their parents prior to the 1870s.[9]

Laws enacted in various forms in both Britain and the United States made families responsible for the support of the aged. While historians have often cited these regulations to prove that families were obligated to care for the aged, careful study of the court records in Britain led

David Thomson to conclude that these laws were, in fact, infrequently enforced and often disregarded.[10] Furthermore, even according to the law, the legal responsibility of the family in Britain was quite limited. Once they married, for instance, daughters had no responsibility for their parents. Men were not responsible for their in-laws, nor were siblings, aunts, uncles, grandchildren, nieces, or nephews legally bound to support aged kin. As well, the courts had to prove that a relative was "of sufficient means" to pay support before any maintenance order could be issued. Similarly, in the United States, Blanche Coll found that officials understood that poor old people usually had poor relatives. Courts occasionally did order people to support an aged parent, but if this order was ignored town officials usually forgot the matter.[11] Rather than forcing a family member to provide for the aged, town officials would reach a mutual agreement in which the responsibility was shared.

Peter Laslett concludes that, in England during the nineteenth century, old people were supported by a wide range of expedients in which family and community collaborated.[12] These findings cause Thomson to assert that, in the case of family support for the aged, statutory provision does not always provide a fair description of standard practice.[13] Instead, when the aged found themselves in need, they turned not to their families but to their community, and the courts, rather than forcing families to provide for the aged, upheld the notion of community or public responsibility for their financial support.[14]

This does not mean that families were not vital to elderly people. While few families were able to provide financial support for their aged kin, children whether married or single played a considerable part in providing care for their parents.[15] In her study of the aged in nineteenth-century Devonshire, Jean Robin found that nine of every ten aged people had at least one unmarried child living with them. Daughters over the age of thirty were particularly evident.[16] Similarly, Michael Anderson found that elderly spinsters in England received a great deal of care and support from kin.[17] These findings are supported by the 1851 census, which revealed that most aged people lived with their children. Various studies of American census reports disclose a similar trend.[18]

Thus, while many government statements from the late nineteenth-century affirm that families were providing less and less care for the aged, it appears that there was no change in the amount of care or attention families provided for the elderly in either Britain or the United States. Instead, what changed was the degree of public assistance distributed to the aged. Once this assistance was reduced, the ability of families to care for the aged was greatly diminished. Public officials, however, refused to acknowledge that it was restrictive relief policies and not uncaring families which caused the noticeable increase in old-age poverty and dependency in the latter decades of the last century.

Historians generally state that the elderly, along with everyone else, suffered at the hands of poor-relief reforms which occurred in both England and the United States during the 1830s. England's infamous Poor Law of 1834, with its authoritarian and restrictive guidelines for providing assistance to the poor and unemployed, has often been cited as an example of the way in which the destitute aged were treated by public poor-relief officials. The image of the workhouse always looms large in most accounts of poor relief in the nineteenth-century.

Yet David Thomson argues that the harsh reforms of 1834 were never enforced, or even intended to be enforced, against the aged. In his study of the Ampthill and Bedford Poor Law Unions, he found little enthusiasm for changes to the Poor Law that thrust responsibility for the aged upon their relatives. The aged, he argues, were relatively unaffected by these legislative changes; indeed, the benevolent attitude exhibited by public officials in earlier periods continued.[19] Despite frequent claims that the Poor Law led to the widespread institutionalization of the aged, Poor Law officials themselves stated that "it is not our intention to issue any such rule" that would force the aged to enter workhouses in order to receive relief.[20] Few aged, in fact, ever did enter workhouses in the nineteenth century.[21]

Similarly, in Philadelphia, as far as the aged were concerned, the idea that institutional aid should completely supplant all other forms of public support was almost always rejected.[22] The overseers of the poor described this proposal as cruel and unfair and said that it made no economic sense. In fact, Blanche Coll discovered evidence that civic officials advocated providing pensions which would keep poor people in their homes. Some even suggested paying family members to care for the aged. As result, although nearly every leading seaport in the American colonies had an almshouse by the 1730s, most aged people were provided with outdoor pensions until at least the middle of the nineteenth century. As late as 1830, less than 10 per cent of public assistance was given in institutions. Even when officials did restrict public relief to institutional aid, as they did in Pennsylvania in 1828, public opinion was so against the idea that outdoor relief was allowed to continue.[23]

The evidence, then, indicates that the aged were not a "social problem" prior to the late nineteenth century. This was not because there were too few of them to constitute a burden. The aged constituted a significant portion of eighteenth- and nineteenth-century populations in England and the United States. A large minority of these people were dependent, yet most were not being supported by kin. Though families and neighbours provided care for the dependent elderly, few relatives were able to maintain them financially. The main reason the aged poor were not a social problem was that the bulk of them were being supported by public poor-relief funds.[24] The aged were treated as a community responsibility and both public opinion and the courts upheld and accepted this situation. While other dependent groups, such as the unemployed, were treated with suspicion by poor-relief officials and often sent to institutions, the aged were generally treated benevolently and permitted to remain within their communities, where they received assistance in their own homes.

This state of affairs was overturned during the final decades of the nineteenth-century, when government officials, in an effort to reduce poor-relief costs, began to restrict both the amount of public assistance being distributed to old people and the amount of public funds expended upon providing them with accommodation. As Raymond Mohl explains, outdoor relief now came under attack virtually everywhere, mainly because of a prolonged economic depression that left far more people dependent upon public assistance than the system could support.[25] Priscilla Clement points out that economic upheavals are always decisive in promoting change to social-welfare policies.[26] The depression hardened attitudes towards the poor and increased the reluctance of officials to expend limited public resources upon relief.

As well, outdoor relief, more than any other poor-relief practice, became the prime target of cost-cutting measures.[27] For instance, in New York during the late nineteenth-century, poor-relief officials found that there was a steadily increasing demand for assistance which a lack of sufficient funds left them totally unable to meet. In response, public outdoor relief was abolished.[28] During the same period, Providence, Rhode Island, slashed outdoor relief expenditures from $150,00 in 1878 to $4,700 two years later.[29]

While such reductions in outdoor relief spending had occurred during earlier periods of economic crisis, such as the 1830s, they had usually been applied only to those deemed "able bodied."[30] After 1870, however, the elimination of outdoor relief was so severe that the aged, "the core of public welfare commitment" and previously the one group left unaffected by restrictive relief policies, were targeted "in a way not seen before or since."[31] In England, the Poor Law budget, the number of elderly people receiving pensions, and the value of the pensions distributed were all halved. Public relief was eliminated for aged people who had relatives capable of maintaining them. Court prosecutions for non-maintenance were increased and the legal concept of family responsibility was extended to include a larger group of relatives. As well, the notion of what constituted "sufficient means" was defined in a manner that left even very poor families liable to support their aged kin.[32] For those who refused to maintain the elderly, the threat of the workhouse was employed.[33]

In a society where the bulk of the aged population was supported by poor-relief payments, such actions could do little else but create a major social crisis.[34] Government policies initiated a huge transfer of responsibility for the support of the aged from the community to the family.[35] In doing so, however, these policies placed upon nineteenth-century families a burden that they were totally unable to bear and so produced widespread poverty and dependency among the aged.[36] Though initiated with the express intent of encouraging family affection, the main impact of the new policies was to increase greatly the workhouse population and remove the aged from their homes.[37] In this sense, the elderly's emergence as a social problem was not the result of irresponsible families. The problem was instead a creation of government.

Government policy in late-nineteenth-century Ontario followed the same pattern. Prior to confederation, most elderly people relied on communal support networks which offered family care as well as the informal assistance of friends and neighbours and the formal support of local government bodies.[38] Over the course of the latter half of the nineteenth century, however, as the provincial government developed the capacities for intervention and regulation,[39] provincial officials used their powers against local relief efforts. As a result, communal support systems were eroded by a series of provincial policy decisions which gradually reduced the power of local communities and officials over social-welfare issues and placed control in the hands of provincial authorities. Provincial welfare policy, rather than encouraging the continuation of communal support systems, focused on replacing these with centralized institutional care. As a cost-cutting measure, the push to place all dependent people within institutions backfired. Within a few decades the demand for institutional care far exceeded the number of available beds and expenditures on institutional care had risen to point that the government decided to reverse its policy and reduce the number of people housed in provincial institutions. It accomplished this by redefining who was eligible for such care in a manner that increased the obligations of families towards the aged.

Traditional histories of social welfare often argued that institutions became necessary because nineteenth-century families were increasingly unwilling to provide care for dependent kin. Institutional administrators regularly complained that many people, especially the aged, were institutionalized because their relatives refused to care for them. In reality, however, late-nineteenth-century families were no less willing to care for their aged than families had been earlier. What changed over the course of the latter half of the century was the amount of care the government expected families to provide.[40] Where once local communities were willing to share responsibility for the aged with families, provincial authorities refused to accept a similar degree of responsibility for the aged.

Upholding the idea that the aged were solely a family responsibility, provincial officials refused to acknowledge that there were limits to the amount of care families could be expected to provided for the aged without some form of assistance. Throughout the late-Victorian era, therefore, there was a steady increase in the level of responsibility Ontarian families were expected to assume for the aged. By the end of the century, families were often forced to shoulder the entire burden of care alone; provincial policies dictated that only in exceptional circumstances were aged people with relatives eligible for public support, which was usually provided in the form of institutional accommodation.

While one could argue that the government was simply unaware of the impact their policies had on families, Eli Zaretsky asserts that governments in England and across North America purposely set out to force families to accept more responsibility for the aged and dependent. He explains that government policies encouraged institutions, not to help families care for those people they found themselves unable to provide for, but to reform families in order to make them more self-sufficient and hence less dependent upon public or communal support.[41] The impulse to place more responsibility for the dependent upon families was part of capitalist society's emphasis on the "self-supporting" family. The middle class of the period cleaved to a "robust individualism" and as a group did its best to ensure that the ideals of self-reliance and independence were embedded not only in state policy but also in the hearts and minds of the working class.[42] As a result, by the late nineteenth century, state policy dictated that individual families should necessarily provide for all the needs of each of their members. Each family, it was felt, should function as an independent unit. Stephanie Coontz explains that communal support networks in which friends and neighbours assisted needy families promoted a form of social interdependence among families that was incompatible with late nineteenth-century middle-class values. That elites and members of the middle class, who directly controlled the making of social policy in the period, generally favoured the establishment of institutions to care for the poor, while farmers and working men preferred the continuation of outdoor relief, suggests that governments did indeed use institutions to promote middle-class notions of the ideal family and its proper role in society.[43]

According to this argument, the provincial government's disdain for outdoor relief was part of a movement against older traditions which encouraged social interdependence among families while its support for institutionalization was inspired by a desire to promote the self-supporting family. Coontz argues that "far from being opposed to the self-supporting family, these institutions arose to buttress it, refusing to let its casualties throw the concept into question or modify its internal arrangements."[44] Institutions were a necessary component of a system which valued self-supporting families since the more the family was expected to fend for itself, rather than being able to rely on the support of their neighbours and community, the more frequently families who were not economically, physically, or emotionally able to provide for all their members required some type of formal public assistance. In the nineteenth-century, this help usually came in the form of an institution which removed from the public eye all those people who could not be cared for by their families.[45]

By encouraging the construction of and use of institutions, the late-nineteenth-century state fostered ideals of individual and familial autonomy. It thereby weakened the primary ties of social interdependence, and signalled the decline of bonds of kinship and community which had been the vital element of communal support networks. Zaretsky concludes that institutions were one means by which the state helped reorganize families and communities, making families increasingly responsible for the welfare and care of those people who could not care for themselves.[46] The available evidence indicates that this is what occurred in Ontario.

Until the last decades of the nineteenth century, most aged people in Ontario who needed public assistance received outdoor relief, which consisted of cash or donations of food, fuel, or clothing given to them in their own home. Prior to 1837, there simply were no institutional modes of relief to turn to. Even many years after that date, only Toronto and Kingston had institutions that accepted the aged and were capable of housing more than a handful of people.[47] Twenty years later, there were still less than twenty private charitable homes and sixty-one public institutions in the province; fifty-three of these were prisons, ten were hospitals, and a further six housed only women and orphans. It was not until the 1880s that institutional care became the standard form of public assistance available for the aged. Nevertheless, the opening of the Toronto House of Industry in 1837 and the Toronto Lunatic Asylum in 1838 marked the first steps in a process that eventually eliminated outdoor relief, emphasized the notion that the aged were properly a familial as opposed to a community responsibility, and forced the aged poor who could not be supported by kin to segregate themselves from their communities in order to receive public assistance.[48]

One of the prime motives behind the initial construction of institutions for the care of the poor and disabled was cost. Starting in the 1830s, massive immigration, combined with economic upheavals, contributed to a substantial rise in the incidence of unemployment and poverty in the province. The cost of providing relief to the masses of needy people escalated beyond the means of the private charity organizations which had previously managed to care for these people.[49] District magistrates also found that they lacked the funds to distribute outdoor relief, such as pensions or grants, to all the aged and needy persons who petitioned them for aid.[50] It was in this environment of fiscal desperation that the provincial government found itself compelled to assume responsibility for the destitute.[51]

The government could have provided financial assistance to private charities and local district and municipal councils, thereby allowing them to continue providing outdoor relief to the poor and to people who were caring for the ill and the aged. Instead, it decided to focus poor-relief efforts on establishing and encouraging the use of institutions. This, Richard Splane elaborates, was largely due to the strength of the movement towards institutional care and away from outdoor relief which was gaining ascendancy on both sides of the Atlantic.[52] At the same time, as the incidence of destitution increased, so did popular distrust of the poor.[53] Since poverty and misfortune were increasingly blamed on personal faults, charity organizations felt that generous assistance would in fact harm the poor for they would take advantage of any assistance that was made too easily available.

It was also believed that the poor needed reform. This reform usually consisted of attempts to instill in them ideals of independence and self-reliance. In most cases, institutions were chosen as the most effective means of implementing such values. As Allan Irving explains, Sir Francis Bond Head had been a strong supporter of the more restrictive aspects of England's 1834 Poor Law reform and, once in Upper Canada as lieutenant governor, he set out to ensure that the same principles – especially the emphasis on institutions – guided the colony's relief practices.[54]

After 1837 the provincial government was able to act upon its belief in institutional care. Private charities increasingly came to rely on government funding and municipal and district councils found themselves unable to cope with the demands for assistance they received. Under these circumstances, the provincial government established an increasing degree of control over public assistance for the poor.[55] As more control over poor-relief policy was placed in the hands of the government, institutions increasingly dominated the poor-relief landscape.

Legislation, such as the 1838 House of Industry Act, vested the responsibility for institutions in the provincial government, thus reducing the influence of local authorities over poor-relief decisions.[56] After 1834 various municipal incorporation acts defined the responsibilities of town councils towards the poor solely in terms of, and in some cases specifically limited the provision of poor relief to, institutional care.[57] In addition, the 1849 Municipal Incorporation Act, while granting some authority relating to poor relief to county councils, restricted municipal powers by putting in question the right of municipalities to tax themselves for the support of the poor.[58] Together, these actions effectively removed control of poor-relief efforts from local authorities and meant that the poor were increasingly subjected to the dictates of provincial policy decisions.[59]

The province, meanwhile, refused to acknowledge any responsibility for outdoor relief even after 1871, when the government had ample revenues to fund such activities.[60] Instead, it chose to limit spending to the construction of provincial institutions, such as asylums, and to assist private charity groups that emphasized institutional care.[61] In fact, the inspector of prisons and public charities, J.W. Langmuir, declared that communal relief systems promoted ineffectual "unsystematic charity." He advocated the elimination of outdoor relief as a means of encouraging the construction of county houses of industry, which he felt should assume the burdens of municipal poor relief.[62] The government formalized its dedication to institutional aid in 1874 with the passing of the Charity Aid Act, which focused provincial funding for private charity organizations on those who provided institutional relief. In a move that put municipal outdoor relief efforts at a distinct disadvantage, provincial assistance was, in most cases, allotted solely on the basis of the number of people resident in any given charitable institution. Even institutions were not eligible to receive funding for any people they decided to assist outside the establishment.[63] As one report noted, "outdoor-relief seems to go for nothing, and the government assistance is given exclusively on the number of permanent paupers assisted. The more permanent these are so much greater the public help!"[64]

The government's bias against outdoor assistance was illustrated by the fact that the Toronto House of Providence, which provided only institutional care, received more than twice as much in provincial subsidies as the Toronto House of Industry, which assisted far more people but provided the bulk of them with outdoor relief.[65] Provincial policies ensured that institutions that attempted to continue distributing both types of poor relief, such as the houses of industry, found themselves, because of financial difficulties, unable to maintain their outdoor-relief

programs as effectively as their institutional care. J.P. Pell of the Toronto St George's Society regularly criticized this aspect of the province's charity policy. He complained that outdoor relief was
"niggardly," mainly because most funding went to institutional care.[66]

This was of particular significance to the aged. One 1879 report declared that, of the applicants for outdoor relief in Toronto, a majority
of the women were beyond middle age and nearly all the men were old
and infirm.[67] It was clear that any reduction in outdoor-relief payments
would affect the aged more severely than anyone else and, as a result,
force more of them than the members of any other group into institutions.

Yet, while provincial policies were increasingly forcing aged people
in need of public assistance to enter institutions, few institutions were
constructed specifically for the elderly. Before the 1890s, there was, in
fact, only limited interest in establishing such institutions. A meeting
held in Toronto in 1883 to investigate erecting an asylum and hospital
for the aged alongside the existing House of Industry was so poorly
attended that the idea was dropped and nothing was done for over a
decade.[68] The result was that the aged were included along with the
deserving poor of all ages, types, and descriptions as the intended residents of the province's houses of industry. As the century progressed,
however, the size of the aged population in Ontario grew rapidly, and
at a much faster rate than the number of beds in public institutions.
Also, specialized facilities were established for other groups, such as
children and women, leaving mainly the elderly in provincial houses of
refuge and county houses of industry.[69] As a consequence of these
trends, most institutions "swiftly found themselves depositaries for the
decaying and the decrepit."[70]

Local authorities, meanwhile, could do little to combat the trend towards institutionalization. Mary Stokes has outlined how municipal
authorities found that, after the passing of the Municipal Corporations
Act or, as it was popularly known, the Baldwin Act in 1849, their autonomy in many areas was reduced. Increasingly, municipalities came
under the power of the central authorities, especially in regard to their
spending. Using the powers granted to them by the Baldwin Act, provincial authorities regularly imposed new responsibilities and, hence,
expenses upon municipal authorities without offering any compensation.[71] This put additional pressure on municipal finances, leaving less
and less money for discretionary spending such as outdoor relief.

With little influence and limited finances, the counties and municipalities of the province found themselves more and more unable to distribute funds within local communities either to help individuals and
families care for those who could not care for themselves or to provide

pensions which enabled people, many of them aged, to remain independent. In Perth, for example, municipal councilmen were claiming that "it would be extremely injudicious" for council to spend "any money that could possibly be avoided."[72] While municipalities never completely halted outdoor-relief payments, evidence indicates that the portion of the population assisted by such funds declined drastically during the last quarter of the century. Since non-institutional relief received no support from provincial authorities, county and municipal councils were forced to seek cost-saving methods of assisting the poor. In this regard, Langmuir and other provincial officials promoted institutional relief as being more effective and less costly than outdoor relief. Reducing municipal poor-relief spending therefore became a strong catalyst for constructing institutions.

Reports of efficiently run institutions saving municipalities money met with interest. In 1877, for example, a debate occurred in Ontario County concerning the benefits of institutional relief for the poor after it was reported that the Wellington County House of Industry cared for its inmates for less than seventy-six cents a week each. Based on this discovery, various municipalities within the county calculated that they could save between $150 and $200 a year on poor relief by sending the poor to an institution instead of providing outdoor relief.[73]

Though some supported the construction of houses of industry because they genuinely believed the poor would be better cared for in an institution, most council members focused their arguments on the possibility that "establishing a Poor House would be a great saving to the county."[74] Almost all the surviving municipal material concerning houses of industry is concerned with the costs of running the institutions, not the quality of care given to the residents. In the counties of Kent, Leeds and Grenville, and Lanark, for instance, most house of industry correspondence was concerned with calculating how much each municipality owed the county council for housing indigents and with expelling paupers from municipalities that did not contribute to the institution's expenses.[75] Caring for the poor became of less importance than ensuring that all "unjust impositions on this charity" were avoided.[76]

Municipalities envisaged institutional relief as a replacement for rather than as a complement to outdoor relief. Frequently, they drastically reduced their spending on outdoor relief once institutional forms of relief were made available. For example, in Brantford, both the county council and the municipal council distributed funds for outdoor poor relief. Yet, once municipal funds were diverted towards maintaining a house of industry, local assistance to groups providing outdoor poor relief was reduced or halted. As the Brantford *Courier* reported, the construction of a house of industry will "remove the Ladies Aid Society from any further responsibility in the matter of charitable donations, at least as far as the city grant is concerned."[77] Once the Ladies Aid Society's municipal grant was eliminated, the group was no longer able to assist the local poor by distributing outdoor relief. As a result, people previously being supported in their own homes were forced to enter the newly constructed House of Industry.

Two investigations of municipal poor relief were carried out in 1874 and 1888. These reports indicated that the number of people assisted by municipal relief declined between the two dates despite the massive population growth experienced in most of the province.[78] In addition, reports of the sums local county councils gave to each pauper during the same period reveal a general trend towards smaller disbursements. While the provincial average for outdoor-relief payments was ten dollars for each person in 1874,[79] after opening a house of industry in 1883 Welland County officials usually granted no more than six dollars in aid to any one person.[80] Other reports suggest that by the 1880s most municipalities distributed between three and eight dollars to each person on their charity list. It also appears that certain councils were less willing to provide aid to people who were caring for others. In Lanark County in 1862, for instance, five people received between twenty and seventy-six dollars each as compensation for caring for indigent or insane individuals.[81] By the 1880s there is little record of similar payments being made. These changes were certainly related to the establishment of county houses of industry, most of which were constructed after 1874. While the information available from newspaper reports and municipal records is far from conclusive, it does suggest that the amounts given as outdoor relief were most likely to decrease in localities which had recently constructed some type of institution to care for the poor.

Lincoln County paid between five and ten dollars a month in outdoor relief to each person on their charity list for the destitute and insane. In this manner, the county council distributed an average of $1,078.65 a year for purposes of outdoor relief between 1882 and 1886. In 1887, however, the council spent only $381 on poor relief and after 1888 spending fell to less than $100 a year.[82] The main reason for this drastic drop in outdoor-relief payments was the opening of the Lincoln County House of Industry in January 1887. Between 1884 and 1887 council was assisting between fourteen and twenty people a year; between 1888 and 1891 it assisted only one (see Table 1). With the opening of a local institution, Lincoln County's recipients of poor relief were cut off from local relief payments and no new names were added to the list.

In effect, the county ceased to distribute outdoor relief once the House of Industry was constructed. Since it was the only source of public assistance available to them after 1887, people requiring support had no choice but to resort to it. While the existing records list most persons entering the institution only as "indigent," Mrs Bowman, Elizabeth Howell, and Mrs Spears, all of whom had been receiving outdoor relief prior to 1887, were listed as having been sent to the House of Industry between January and June 1887.[83] It is likely that several of the other "indigents" were also people formerly on the outdoor-relief list.

The House of Industry was expensive to build, but its daily maintenance did not cost the county much more than had previously been spent on outdoor relief. It also allowed the county to support a few more people: according to the 1891 census, the institution had twenty-one inmates. While the province limited the amount the county could spend on outdoor relief by refusing to offer provincial grants for such activities, the county did receive a $4,000 legislative grant in 1891 to assist with the expenses of maintaining the poor in an institution.[84] Financially, institutionalizing the poor made a great deal of sense for Lincoln County. The records are silent, however, on the quality of care people received in an institution that was constructed specifically to save money.

While information in other counties is inconclusive, it seems likely that most counties did as Lincoln and built institutions, not as a means of supplementing their poor-relief efforts, but as a replacement for all other forms of assistance. In Brockville, for example, the debate over the establishment a local house of industry centred upon whether the poor would be better served by the county spending its money on an institution or by distributing grants to various charities which provided outdoor relief. It does not appear that the idea of supporting both forms of relief was discussed.[85]

As municipalities provided less assistance for the non-institutionalized poor, it grew increasingly difficult for aged persons to remain in their own homes and for other people to provide care for them. As a result, outdoor relief became a less and less viable means of support for the aged.[86] This process was exacerbated by the fact that the immediate impact of the government's refusal to recognize outdoor relief as a legitimate subject of provincial support was to encourage the construction of new institutions at the expense of communal relief systems at the local level. There were only four publicly assisted charity establishments in 1866, but there were thirty-three such facilities in 1893. By the end of the century this number had risen to nearly one hundred.[87] Since municipalities reduced or even eliminated their outdoor-relief efforts once an institution was established nearby, each additional insti-

Table 1
Outdoor-relief payments in Lincoln County, 1882–91

Recipient	1882		1883		1884		1885		1886		1887		1888	1889	1890	1891
	Jan.	June	Jan.	June	Jan.	June	Jan.	June	Jan.	June	Jan.	June				

Terryberry
Caugh
Shelley
Isaubacker
Burghart
Gregory
Howell
Simmerman
Bowmann
Spears
Cook
Wilcox
Finn
Wilkinson
Dolan
Melow
Slough
Turl
Schwabb
Osbourne

— = length of time person received outdoor relief

* = died

Source: AO, RG 21, Municipal Records, Lincoln County Clerk Treasurer's Letterbook (see expenses for insane and destitute), 1884–91

tution led to a further reduction in the amount of outdoor assistance available to the aged poor and their families. Basically, the insistence, on the part of the provincial government, on directing all public funds to institutional care effectively eliminated outdoor relief, a major component of most communal support systems, as an option for anyone needing more than immediate temporary aid.[88] The disappearance of outdoor aid forced many persons who required long-term assistance, which was often the case with the elderly, to enter an institution.

It is certain that many people, the aged in particular, often required institutional care. Some, such as the senile, could often not be cared for within their communities. Nevertheless, numerous other old people could have lived independently while others who could not live on their own could have been cared for by their families, if only the government had chosen to make financial support available to them. Few governments, however, pursued such alternatives. In most jurisdictions, the results of government support for institutional care were similar. David Thomson discovered that in England the availability of outdoor relief had a large impact on rates of institutionalization. As the incidence of outdoor relief declined, institutionalization increased.[89] Michael Anderson attributes increasing rates of institutionalization among the aged in Cambridgeshire after 1871 to the implementation of an anti-outdoor-relief policy.[90] During this same period, Jill Quadagno reports that poor-relief officials tried to reduce outdoor-relief expenses by deciding that old people should not live alone. People over the age of seventy who lived independently were cut off from outdoor relief and sent to the workhouse unless they went to live with family or friends.[91]

While anti-outdoor-relief policies in Ontario were not as brutally enforced as those in England, the refusal of the provincial government to assist people outside institutions still forced numerous aged people to enter houses of industry, houses of refuge, and old age homes. Insisting that institutions were the only way to provide public assistance to the needy increased the number of people requiring institutional care by eliminating other viable options.[92] It also created undue hardships for many poor people and their families because, while the provincial policies eliminated most alternative forms of relief, the government failed to provide sufficient institutional facilities to accommodate all the people who needed care.

While government policies directed all those in need of assistance towards institutions, the province did little more than encourage counties to provide adequate facilities to accommodate all those in need. Often, outdoor relief was eliminated before anyone could ensure that the people who had formerly been assisted in this manner could be housed in an institution. In some municipalities, outdoor relief was limited to people requiring temporary or emergency assistance before a house of industry had been erected to care for those individuals who needed more long-term support.[93] Once again this problem developed largely because of provincial funding policies. While the province agreed to assist establishments that provided institutional care for the poor, it did not, until 1890, provide funds to assist counties with the cost of constructing institutions. Although houses of industry saved counties money in the long run, they were usually expensive to construct. Lincoln County, for example, spent almost $28,000 over a four-year period to construct and prepare its house of industry to receive residents.[94] This deterred many counties from establishing a house of industry, while others reduced outdoor-relief expenditures in order to accumulate funds with which to commence constructing an institution. The overall effect of these trends was that there was never anywhere near the number of beds required to accommodate all the aged people who needed care.[95] This forced the institutions that did exist to adopt rather rigid entrance requirements and to refuse entry to anyone who did not meet the specifications.[96]

Despite restrictive admission policies, the aged came to constitute an ever increasing segment of the province's institutional population. This was mainly because provincial policies left elderly people with nowhere else to go. Forcing the aged into institutions, however, had far more serious consequences than merely removing the aged from their homes and segregating them from their communities. The institutionalization of the aged population affected not only how the aged lived but also how they were perceived by institution administrators, government officials, and the public in general. Institutions focused their attention on the desperate and needy elderly, an approach that made the most decrepit and dependent segment of the aged population the most visible.[97] This both created and confirmed the image of the elderly as incapacitated, unproductive, and helpless.[98] Often, officials and administrators implemented policies towards the aged based on this impression. Such policies, which tended to have a significant impact on the future of many aged people and their families, rarely bore any relation to the experience and situation of the vast majority of the aged population which resided outside of institutions. However, government officials, who tended to formulate policies based on what was visible to them, seldom saw the vast number of non-institutionalized aged people in one place at one time. They saw only the elderly who filled the rooms and corridors of the province's houses of industry and homes of refuge.

When one looked only at the institutionalized aged, it did appear that a large portion of the aged population was destitute and without families able or at least willing to care for them. Despite attempts to limit the number of aged people admitted into institutions, both the number of aged people within their walls and the portion of the institutionalized population they represented grew steadily during the final decades of the nineteenth century. Indeed, it appeared to officials that there was no end to the number of aged people who needed public care. The main explanation they could find for this state of affairs was that families and communities were using institutions as a means of evading their obligations towards the aged.

There was a certain logic to the view that families were institutionalizing the aged at a steadily increasing rate during the 1890s. At the beginning of the decade, the elderly formed a minority of the population within institutions. By the end of the decade, however, the number of old people in institutions had grown and these people had come to form a large portion of the province's institutionalized population. The fact that the institutionalized elderly population was increasing during a period when the government was building more institutions, many specifically designed to shelter aged people, added further weight to the government's argument.

Yet the truth was more complex. Census reports indicate that in 1891 there were 152,488 persons in Ontario who were over the age of sixty. In September of the same year, the inspector of prisons and public charities reported that there were 1,260 beds available in government-funded charitable institutions which were likely occupied by aged people.[99] In addition, there were some 3,318 beds in the various provincial asylums for the insane. This provided potential accommodation for a total of 4,478 aged persons. Even if every one of these beds had been occupied by someone over the aged of sixty, this number would have represented only 3.5 per cent of the province's total aged population.

In reality, moreover, the number of elderly people in these institutions was much smaller. For instance, at no time did the aged constitute more than 20 per cent of the insane asylum population. In fact, between 1888 and 1896, the elderly comprised only 15 per cent of the total number of people admitted to all provincial asylums.[100] Also, as the table below demonstrates, an 1889 investigation indicated that aged people accounted for less than half of the residents of the province's county houses of industry[101] (see Table 2). This meant that the old people in Ontario's institutions in 1891 represented no more than 2 per cent of the total aged population of the province.

Over the course of the 1890s, the aged population within public institutions grew to the point that by the turn of the century the elderly constituted approximately 80 per cent of the population of Ontario's houses of refuge and 70 per cent of its county houses of industry.[102]

Table 2
Number of aged people reported as resident in houses of industry in Ontario, 1889

County House of Industry	Total Inmates	Aged Inmates	Percentage Aged
Brant	60	unknown*	unknown*
Elgin	109	46	42.2%
Lincoln	52	19	36.6%
Norfolk	75	19	25.3%
Middlesex	127	60	47.2%
Waterloo	118	72	61.1%
Welland	59	35	59.3%
Wellington	77	54	70.1%
York	157	78	49.7%
Total	774*	383	49.4%

* Brant was not included in the total calculations.
Source: *Ontario Sessional Paper*, no. 61 (1889).

This occurred even though the decade was a period of institution building. The number of houses of refuge, county houses of industry, and other publicly funded charitable institutions in the province increased from sixty-two at the beginning of the decade to nearly one hundred in 1901. In houses of refuge alone, the number of beds almost doubled, increasing from 1,260 to 2,268 (see Table 3). In total, provincial institutions could accommodate as many as 4,485 persons by the end of the century.[103] At the same time, almost 2,000 new beds were added to provincial asylums for the insane. In all, this represented an 80 per cent increase in the number of aged people who could be potentially housed in a public institution. When the aged population of these institutions grew despite their enlarged capacity it is not surprising that government officials would conclude, at least initially, that the aged were being sent to institutions at an ever increasing rate and that the burden on the public treasury would soon become unbearable. The truth was that this was not the case.

The newly provided accommodations in provincial institutions came nowhere near keeping pace with the even more dramatic increase in the total number of aged people in the province. Between 1891 and 1901 the number of people over the age of sixty grew by over 30,000 to a total of 182,735. The result of this growth was that, even though the number of beds in provincial institutions increased during the 1890s,

Table 3
Number of beds available in Ontario's houses of refuge, 1889–99

Year	Total Number of Beds
1889	1,260
1891	1,349
1893	1,706
1895	1,917
1897	2,120
1899	2,268

Source: AR (1889–99), "Report of the Inspector of Prisons and Public Charities upon Houses of Refuge."

these institutions could still shelter no more than 3 per cent of Ontario's aged population. Thus, while officials blamed the ever increasing numbers of old people in public institutions on the increasing willingness of families to abandon the aged, in fact the portion of the total aged population being sent to institutions changed little between 1891 and 1901. Despite government reports, even if the aged had filled every bed in every institution, the vast majority of them would never have seen the inside of one of these places. A rough estimate indicates that, for every aged individual in an institution, there were at least thirty-three others being cared for by kin or living on their own.

This situation was not unique. Various studies have confirmed that, during the nineteenth century, the institutionalized aged population across North America never formed more than 3 to 5 per cent of the total number of people over the age of sixty. Carole Haber, for example, argues that in 1904 up to 98 per cent of the aged population of Massachusetts lived outside state institutions.[104] Barbara Rosencrantz and Maris Vinovskis demonstrate that only a very small portion of the aged insane were ever placed in asylums. They conclude that, despite the rising numbers of aged people in asylums, the aged were still the least likely of all insane people to be institutionalized.[105] Similar conclusions have been reached by Brian Gratton[106] in his study of the aged in Boston, and by David Thomson in an analysis of the institutionalized population of nineteenth-century England.[107]

Nevertheless, like their counterparts a century later, Ontario officials maintained that aged people were being institutionalized needlessly. They argued that "the number of aged and infirm people who can work very little or not at all is not a large one. The number of those of this class who have no friends to support them," and hence may become candidates for institutionalization, "is still smaller."[108] While this may have been true, the government assumed that anyone who had "friends," a term that referred to relatives as well as non-related people, was not a candidate for institutionalization. Thus, even the minority of the aged population who sought the shelter of institutions because they truly needed assistance often found that restrictive admission polices denied them access to care. One observer commented that it was often so difficult to obtain admission to a house of industry that it "was easier for an aged infirm pauper to get into jail than into [an] institution."[109]

It was common for institutions to adopt policies that denied access to institutions to any person from outside the region served by the establishment. The Toronto House of Industry declared that "the managers of this institution have unanimously resolved that in the future all cases coming from other municipalities be refused admission."[110] This left people who lived in counties lacking a house of industry with no place to go. Institutions also demanded that residents be easy to care for and that they behave appropriately. These requirements affected the aged more severely than others because they frequently suffered from illnesses or senility which made them difficult to care for or troublesome. As one house of industry inspector pointed out, the aged residents were "in many cases most trying patients."[111]

Institution officials sometimes ejected "troublesome" inmates once their behaviour caused them to become a nuisance or they required medical attention that was beyond the usually limited capabilities of the establishment.[112] This was especially true in cases of pronounced senility. It was frequently reported that other inmates were disturbed by the "gibbering idiots."[113] One eighty-year-old woman had been living in a house of industry for several years. Once she became demented, however, she was sent to an insane asylum since the attendants claimed that they could no longer manage her. Similar reasons regularly prompted the sisters of the Kingston House of Providence to transfer old women who became abusive or violent to the Rockwood Asylum for the Insane.[114] Gerald Grobb adds that financial considerations often underlay such actions. While an aged person remained in a local institution their care was payed for by municipal funds; once they were labelled senile they could be sent to an asylum where provincial dollars would pay for their care.[115]

It was the aged with kin, however, who suffered the most from limitations on the number of elderly persons eligible for institutional care. Institutional administrators increasingly began to express the view that the aged were not proper candidates for institutions. Instead, it was argued, they should be cared for by their families.[116] Reflecting the new emphasis on the self-supporting family and the increased responsibility for dependent kin that late nineteenth-century society vested in families, officials argued that the making accessible of public shelters would "take away ... the filial obligation for the support of aged parents which is the main bond of family solidarity."[117]

Of course, the very economic crisis that was causing bureaucrats to advocate cost-cutting measures was also having a major impact upon the working class. As David and Rosemary Gagan explain, during the 1890's working-class incomes and standards of living fell, causing individual and familial distress.[118] The government itself reported in 1895 that, "owing to the general depression in business and consequent hard times during the past years, the number of paupers has greatly increased."[119] These deteriorating economic conditions certainly affected the ability of families to care for dependent relatives.

Yet the government was blind to this reality. Legislators and bureaucrats rarely understood that many families, especially among the working class, lacked the physical or financial resources required to care for an aged relative. For the most part, politicians and officials belonged to the elite and tended to base their image of family care on the situation found in their own homes. They thought in terms of a large family that was able to "easily manage" the care of an infirm, ill, or senile older person because of the presence of several kin in the household. As Michael Katz pointed out in his study of nineteenth-century Hamilton, however, only the wealthy could afford large households.[120] Also, unlike the majority of the population, the wealthy were able to provide care for ill kin without worrying about the financial strain such actions might place upon the family.

It also appears that, because of its lack of political power, the working class could be effectively ignored by bureaucrats and legislators alike. Universal manhood suffrage was a fairly recent innovation in Ontario, Oliver Mowat having introduced the reform in 1888, and for many years it had only a minimal impact on the political landscape. The Knights of Labour attempted to elect working-class men to the legislature to ensure that the government would "take some interest in the welfare of the class,"[121] but the movement was organized in only a few locations and its success was modest to put it mildly. By 1894 the Knights were described as "devastated."[122] While their activities and those of other working-class groups forced Conservatives and Liberals alike to pass certain pieces of labour legislation, they achieved little with regard to improvements in social policy or social spending.

Ignoring both the circumstances and the needs of the dependent elderly and their working-class families, the government instead pursued policies that were more in line with views of middle-class reformers. In almost all of their activities, these reformers displayed a distinct lack of understanding of or sympathy for the poor. When working-class families failed to live up to middle-class notions of acceptable behaviour or to carry out what reformers felt were their proper responsibilities and obligations, the reformers, instead of reconsidering their assumptions, advocated the use of state intervention to force the lower classes to conform to their ideals.[123]

In the realm of caregiving for the dependent aged, government policy makers appear to have accepted the basic premise of the reformers' arguments, perhaps because it was a convenient justification for cost-cutting measures. Social spending, which represented 32.4 per cent of provincial expenditures in 1893, made up only 14.7 per cent of spending by 1911.[124] Since over 70 per cent of the social-welfare budget consisted of expenditures on institutions, especially mental hospitals and government-funded charitable institutions such as county houses of industry and houses of refuge, these cuts could not help but affect the availability and quality of institutional care for the aged. To justify them, the government argued that it would be better for everyone if families carried a larger share of the burden. In making this demand upon families, however, the state was enforcing a notion of the ideal family that was completely beyond the capacities of most of the families that would be affected by government social policies or institutional regulations. It was also based upon a distorted image of the past.

The assertion that the aged were institutionalized mainly because their families were neglecting them rested on the false assumption that families had cared for the aged in the past and, therefore, had no reason for not continuing to do so. While in earlier decades the aged had indeed been cared for at home, that care was not necessarily provided by the family exclusively. Officials also neglected to consider the fact that, by the end of the nineteenth century, the communal support networks which had supported families in their efforts to care for their aged kin had been undermined by provincial policy. The informal assistance of neighbours and friends never disappeared completely, but the formal support of local governments that was vital to communal relief systems had become negligible. As a result, families were usually forced to provide all the necessary care by themselves in a way that they had rarely been forced to do in the past. Nevertheless, the assumption that families had once cared for the aged on their own and could therefore do so again caused some institutions to refuse aged people access to their establishments. They did so without offering any alternative forms of assistance to the aged or the families who were expected to care for them, an approach that had tragic consequences for many aged people and their families.

It is true that most aged inmates of houses of industry had no family. In Wellington County, for example, the elderly females in the House of Industry "shared a paucity of kin."[125] This finding has been confirmed by several studies of public institutions across North America and Britain. Michael Katz concluded that a lack of children, "more than any other factor, led to an aged person's institutionalization."[126] Yet historians often ignore the fact that by the 1890s only people with no kin to support them were normally permitted into institutions. This meant that aged people with kin suffered the consequences of the ideology of the self-supporting family by being denied access to public institutions solely on the basis of their having living relatives. The majority of the institutionalized aged people who did have relatives came from families who were simply too poor to feed them,[127] but increasingly even poverty did not exempt people from the burden of caring for their aged kin.[128]

In the name of familial responsibilities, institution officials often tried to locate relatives in order to force them to take responsibility for their aged kin. Often when relatives were discovered, inmates were discharged into their care since they were no longer seen to be fit candidates for public charity. This was the case with one destitute old woman in Ottawa who had found refuge in the Protestant Orphan's Home. As Lorna McLean recounts, the woman had lived in the home for one year when it was discovered that she had two sons to support her. She was dismissed and sent to her children.[129] Unlike communal support networks, which recognized that families were not always able to care for an aged relative without community assistance, institutional caregivers demanded that families care for their aged regardless of their financial ability. These tactics ignored the fact that, if a person's relatives were able or willing to provide care, he or she would probably not have arrived in the institution to begin with.

By limiting municipal outdoor relief for the poor and aged, therefore, provincial policies reduced the effectiveness of the communal support networks which had accompanied this formal relief system. Institutional care was established to replace community relief but various fiscal restraints, combined with ideological concerns about familial responsibilities, prevented many needy aged people from gaining access to institutions. They were thus left dependent on relatives who were totally unable to care for them. In short, the combination of the province's preference for institutional care and the emergence of an ideology that emphasized the self-supporting family deprived large numbers of elderly of any form of support. Casualties of "the great social transformation," they usually found themselves destitute and homeless. As one late-nineteenth-century Canadian commentator noted, "we build large buildings to accommodate unfortunates, but we initiate no system whereby the aged and the needy will be able to live without begging."[130]

When begging failed, many homeless old people found themselves imprisoned in local jails. Nineteenth-century laws in Ontario permitted county magistrates to confine homeless old people in the local jail as vagrants. While in earlier decades the aged had formed only a small portion of jail inmates, by the later decades of the century their numbers were significant. The increase in the number of old people in jails was almost certainly a direct consequence of state policy. The aged poor simply had nowhere else to go. As one jail official noted: "I am led to believe that in many cases these old people are placed in gaol simply because it is cheaper for the counties thus to maintain them than to provide a respectable place for their care."[131] It was not until 1899 that the inspector of prisons and public charities could state that the "County Homes which have been established of late for the care of old dependent people have materially relieved the crowding of our gaol by old people committed under the Vagrancy Act."[132]

Even prisons would accept the aged only as long as they were not senile or hard to manage. As with houses of industry, the presence of anyone who disrupted the daily routine or disturbed the other prisoners was not tolerated. From the 1830s, when the Niagara Quarter Sessions was told that one old man had to be removed from the local jail since he was "a great annoyance" to the other prisoners, to the 1890s, when jail inspectors noted that senile and unruly inmates were "very annoying to those in charge on account of the extra care" they required, the aged were frequently ejected from jails.[133] Once the facilities were available, these individuals would normally be sent to an asylum for the insane.

CONCLUSION

In the 1890s, determining the boundary between state responsibilities and family obligations towards the aged became a key element in provincial policies concerning the institutionalization and support of Ontario's elderly people. Basically, the government faced a problem similar to the one confronting the province's legislators today: how should society deal with a rapid increase in the demand for institutional accommodation for the aged during a period of fiscal restraint? The nineteenth-century answer was to blame the situation on the irresponsibility of families. The government insisted that the increasing number of aged people in institutions was obvious evidence that families were shirking their duties and attempting to force upon the state responsibilities which properly belonged to the family. In response, the government simply restricted the admission of old people to institutions and declared that the care of the aged was a family obligation. In defining the boundaries between family obligations and state responsibilities in this manner, the Ontario government argued that, prior to the creation of provincially funded institutions, the aged were the sole responsibility of their families. It was not unreasonable, therefore, in a time of fiscal crisis, for the state to request that families once again assume the responsibilities that they had formerly carried out.

In reality, the provincial government was doing more than merely returning to the family responsibilities that it had previously discharged. Traditionally, rather than being solely a family responsibility, the aged had been viewed as a legitimate concern of the entire community. Friends, neighbours, and members of the community in general assisted families in the performance of their caring functions. This chapter has demonstrated that, when the Ontario government argued that the care of the aged was the obligation of the family, it was in fact attempting to redefine the boundary between state responsibilities and family obligations in a way that placed a far greater share of responsibility upon the family than had previously been the case.

Defining the care of the aged in this fashion, however, allowed the government to justify its refusal to increase public expenditures on institutional accommodation for the dependent aged. Promoting an image of families as irresponsible and uncaring generated sympathy for policies that were really intended to reduce the state's responsibility for the poor and thereby reduce social-welfare spending.

Institutions and the Impact of Public Policy on the Aged: The Elderly Patients of Rockwood Asylum, 1866–1906

At the end of the nineteenth century, institutionalization rates in Ontario were soaring and the cost of constructing and maintaining public institutions for the indigent was rising steeply. Within these institutions the growth of the aged segment of the population was particularly acute. The Ontario government, accordingly, sought to save itself money by halting the tide of institutionalization, especially among the aged. One way it attempted to do this was to shame families into taking on a greater share of responsibility for the dependent elderly. As a result, numerous public statements were made concerning the degree to which families were heartlessly abandoning their elderly in institutions. Nowhere is the attitude underlying these statements more obvious than in the records of Ontario's provincial asylums for the insane. Nineteenth-century medical superintendents of various provincial asylums argued that, rather than having legitimate reasons for placing aged relatives in an asylum, families merely used the institutions as a "convenient place to get rid of inconvenient people."[1]

In the view of most of the province's insane asylum administrators, most of the old people sent to the asylums were not insane but merely suffering from the ravages of senility. As the inspector of the Hamilton asylum reported in 1899, "many [patients] are old people suffering from mental senility; the family may be unable to provide the means of caring for them. They are sent to the asylum simply for safe keeping and to ease the burden upon the friends."[2] Within an asylum, senile aged persons were labelled as chronic cases who could not be treated and would never recover. Moreover, since asylums administrators felt that their prime mission was treatment, few institutions willingly admitted incurable cases.[3] It was argued that the asylum was not a "place for the relatives of senile dementi to place their unfortunate under our care."[4] One asylum superintendent was "outraged" by the common practice of committing harmless old persons. He claimed that "cases of purely senile dementia should not be properly numbered among the insane."[5] These people, it was reported, arrived at the institution not because they required care but "through the importunity of their friends."[6] The admission of feeble and senile individuals, so officials maintained, reduced the number of recoveries asylum doctors could produce and as a result kept the institutions from performing their proper functions.[7]

Nevertheless, as the number of elderly people in the overall population grew, the admission of senile old people into asylums increased. Asylum superintendents began to fear that mental institutions would fill to capacity with the incurable and the unwanted. As one administrator lamented, the asylum "is no longer a hospital for the insane, but a veritable 'Home for Incurables.'"[8] More important, officials questioned whether asylum funds could be properly used to maintain chronic cases since the care of these people was, by 1897, becoming "an enormous tax upon the state."[9] As the medical superintendent of the Hamilton asylum reported, "a great difference of opinion has existed in regard to the best method of caring for the chronic insane, chiefly from an economic standpoint."[10] As far as the admission of senile old people was concerned, it was believed that the "very liberality of the Government in providing such ample accommodation at cheap rates, or even free, acts as a powerful stimulus in deciding to transfer the burden from the home to the state."[11] It was asserted that government was being called upon, with increasing frequency, to assume burdens which, "in all fairness, should be carried by the people."[12]

Being both alarmed and dismayed at what they felt was the unacceptable size of the elderly population within institutions, asylum administrators began to advocate admission policies which insisted that "until homes and refuges for aged people become generally established, the applications to admit victims of senility should be severely discouraged."[13] Family situation, it seems, played a large role in determining whether an aged person was defined as senile or insane and therefore eligible for asylum treatment. Authorities were more willing to accept someone labelled as insane if that person had no relatives.[14] When an aged patient had a family, that patient would usually be classified as being "merely senile" regardless of the behaviour he or she exhibited, since it was assumed that families should be responsible for their aged kin.[15] Thus, at the very point when the aged population was growing and their families experienced an increasing need for the services of the province's insane asylums, the hospitals, in an attempt to reduce costs by placing a greater portion of the burden of care for the aged upon their families, were endeavouring to restrict the aged's access to institutions.

It was common for asylum superintendents to blame the rising number of aged admissions on a declining sense of familial responsibility. When asylums officials decided that they had to limit the number of aged people admitted into mental institutions, they frequently used the ideal of the self-supporting family to justify their claims that the aged, rather than being placed in asylums, should be cared for at home by relatives. It was argued that families admitted their aged kin to institutions merely because they did not want to be bothered caring for them themselves. In England and across North America, asylum superintendents began to report that "there is not excuse whatsoever for their [the elderly's] commitment – and it can be explained only on the basis of a loosening of natural family ties and a desire to be relieved of dutiful responsibilities."[16]

The Pennsylvania Board of Charities reiterated a common sentiment among institutional authorities when it reported that most aged people, "selfishly neglected by those who owe them everything," "are thrust into seclusion in order that they may not be burdens, and too frequently forgotten by those through whose veins flows the same blood. They must helplessly and hopelessly wait, receiving kindness and care from those who are neither kith nor kin."[17] Children, it was believed, were merely "unwilling to inconvenience themselves" and only too willingly "shirked their duties" by sending their "troublesome" parents away once they had become an "encumbrance" upon the family.[18] It was also argued that this growing willingness of families to institutionalize the aged meant that, by the final decades of the century, the aged were more likely to end up in an asylum than they ever had been. Government officials reported that "there is a disposition among all classes now not to bear with the trouble that may arise in their own homes. If a person is troublesome from senile dementia, dirty in his habits, they will not bear with it now. Persons are more easily removed to an asylum than they were a few years ago."[19]

In Ontario, one asylum superintendent stated that the senile were admitted merely because "the condition necessitates a certain amount of attention on the part of friends, and this I am forced to admit seems to be the cause of committal."[20] It was claimed by officials that these "ancient and senile adults, whose only crime was to become a burden," could have been cared for "as well, if not better at home."[21] Yet, asylum inspectors reported, there was a growing tendency among the relatives of the senile to "foist them upon the Government."[22] Despite the demographic facts, the increase in elderly admissions to insane asylums was attributed to a growing indifference on the part of families towards their aged kin, rather than to a genuine increase in the number of old people in need of specialized medical care. Also, while various explanations were presented as to why families were becoming so irresponsible, no one acknowledged that various government and institutional policies played a large role in forcing families to send aged people to asylums, since such facilities were the only alternative left to them.

These various themes are central to the story of the Rockwood Asylum for the Insane in Kingston. Though established in 1858 as a hospital for the province's criminally insane, as early as 1862 it was said to house not only the "criminal class" but "lunatics of every description."[23] After confederation, Rockwood became a federal concern but it was returned to provincial control in 1872. Private mental hospitals never housed more than a fraction of Ontario's insane during the nineteenth century. Rockwood, as one of the larger mental institutions, accounted for between 12 and 20 per cent of the province's total insane asylum population in any given year. On average, the hospital contained 13.8 per cent of Ontario's institutionalized insane. Between its opening and 1907, a total of 4,204 patients,[24] who were in most years evenly divided between males and females, were treated at Rockwood.[25] Of these, a total of 315, or 7.4 per cent of all cases studied, were at least sixty years of age.[26] The average age was sixty-eight, but many of these inmates were over eighty and at least one was over ninety.

The numbers cited here do not include patients who, while they may have been elderly, had been admitted to the institution at a much earlier age. For the purposes of this study the term "aged patients" refers only to those people who were admitted to the asylum when they were over the age of sixty. Asylum officials would often cite the number of aged people who died in the asylum in any given year, which included all aged people in the asylum regardless of when they had been admitted, even though it was clear that people who were admitted when they were actually over the age of sixty often formed a minority of these deaths. In this manner, however, officials could provide the public with an inflated impression of the degree to which the aged were over-populating asylums. For instance, in 1893 almost all of the aged people who died in the Toronto asylum had been admitted to the institution when they were middle-aged or younger. One sixty-eight-year-old man had been there for forty-five years.[27] While these people may have been in the asylum when over the age of sixty, they were admitted to the asylum before they reached that age. Hence, one cannot justifiably use these people as a source of information concerning the admissions of the aged into institutions.

The admissions of elderly people to Rockwood were not constant. Both the number of aged in the asylum and the portion of the institu-

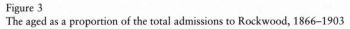

Figure 3
The aged as a proportion of the total admissions to Rockwood, 1866–1903

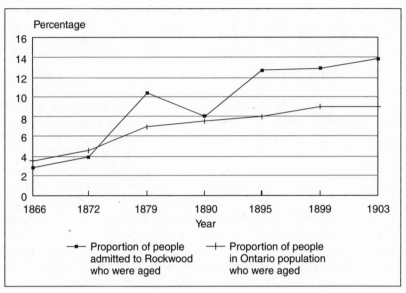

tion's population they represented changed over time. There were no aged persons admitted to Rockwood before 1866 and, until 1881, there were rarely more than two or three people over the age of sixty admitted in any given year. In total, during the first twenty-three years of operation, thirty-six elderly persons were sent to the asylum. In the next sixteen years, however, 205 aged people were admitted. While the aged never formed more than 3 per cent of the total admissions before 1879, they composed over 12 per cent of the new arrivals in 1895 and almost 14 per cent by 1903. (See Figure 3.) Given that the aged formed 3.1 per cent of the total population of the province in 1851, 7.2 per cent by 1891, and 8.4 per cent by 1901, it appears that over the course of the century the aged came to represent a portion of the insane-asylum admissions than was increasingly greater than their demographic presence in the overall population would seemingly justify.

Nevertheless, the actual portion of the total aged population found inside insane asylums changed little between 1866 and 1906. This can be explained by the fact that, while the aged portion of the asylum admissions changed dramatically over the years, the increase in the actual number of patients involved was small. For instance, while the aged's share of Rockwood's admissions grew from 3 to 14 per cent between 1866 and 1906 (most of the growth took place after 1890), the resulting increase in the aged population of the asylum was not significant.

Table 4
Aged asylum population compared to the total population of Rockwood

Year	Total Asylum Population	Number of Aged Residents	Aged as % of Total
1887	681	56	8.2%
1890	674	56	8.3%
1895	565	54	9.6%
1897		64	
1899	558	46	8.2%

Source: AR (1887–99) and also AO, RG 10, series 20–F–1 case files.

This group grew from two aged people in 1866 to a maximum of sixty-four between that date and 1901. Thus, the apparently alarming 11 per cent increase in the portion of the asylums admissions who were aged led to the addition of only sixty-two elderly residents to the asylum population. (See Table 4.) This pattern was similar throughout the various provincial asylums. At the same time, the seemingly small increase in the aged portion of the total provincial population, from 7.2 per cent in 1891 to 8.4 per cent in 1901, masked the fact that the aged population actually increased by 30,000 people. Against this background, it is clear that although the aged were indeed more visible inside mental hospitals, a steadily larger segment of the total elderly population existed outside institutions.

All that said, the argument that families were abandoning the aged in institutions in ever increasing numbers was promoted by the fact that, once admitted to the asylum, few aged people left alive. Only one-quarter of the aged people admitted to Rockwood were eventually discharged. Most of these discharges occurred around the turn of the century, when hospital administrators were hesitant to admit and reluctant to retain chronically ill elderly patients. The bulk of the aged people who arrived at Rockwood remained there until they died (58 per cent) or were transferred to another asylum (18 per cent), where most eventually died. (See Figure 4.)

Considering that the aged comprised an ever increasing portion of the patients admitted to Rockwood and, as a result, made up a greater portion of the total asylum population, and that once inside the institution most aged people remained until they died, it is easy to see why asylum officials argued that many families were refusing to care for their elderly members. It is also easy to understand why some histori-

Figure 4
Fate of aged people admitted to Rockwood

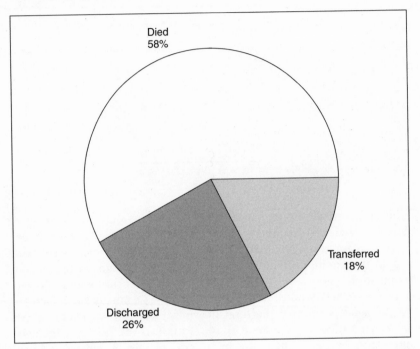

Died
58%

Transferred
18%

Discharged
26%

ans have accepted these officials' arguments. Andrew Scull argues that the increase in aged admissions to asylums during the latter decades of the nineteenth century was due to the fact that, as asylums became more common, the stigma attached to consigning burdensome relatives to asylums evaporated along with any sense of remorse over abandoning familial and kinship obligations.[28] Similarly, Richard Fox has claimed that families committed the aged to asylums because it was a convenient way to rid themselves of the burden of accommodating persons who had become bothersome and who were unable to contribute their share to the family production.[29] These arguments, however, take the official reports of asylum administrators and the various statistics they produced in defence of their statements at face value.

Fortunately, insane asylums produced far more complete records than most provincial institutions. Aside from recording general operational details, asylums kept detailed patient records. The information in these case files reveals that few families committed their aged members to the asylum by choice: most did so out of necessity. These records also suggest that, when aged people were refused admission to an asylum as a means of encouraging or forcing their families to care for them, on the assumption that they would be better cared for by kin, both the aged and their families suffered.

There were some harmless patients who really did not need to be placed in an asylum. A small number were in fact abandoned by relatives who just did not want the responsibility of caring for an elderly person and found the institution to be a convenient place to dump "granny." For instance, in 1885, a sixty-five-year-old woman with five children and a husband was sent to the Rockwood asylum from the Toronto Asylum for the Insane where she had been confined after having been found living alone in the forest. She commented that she liked the asylum better than the bush.[30] Similarly, a sixty-four-year-old man was sent to the asylum from a jail. When he died in 1906 his remains had to be buried by the asylum. Although he reportedly had six living children, his family made no attempt to contact the institution or claim his body. Another woman was placed in the institution by her family in 1895. They never contacted her or the asylum again.

As disheartening as these cases may have been, they were exceptional. Most "harmless" individuals, rather than being abandoned, were people who simply had no relatives to care for them. Many were found homeless. One eighty-year-old woman had been jailed as a vagrant. She was sent to a house of industry but was returned to jail because she swore and was unmanageable. Finally, she was sent to the asylum where, upon arrival, she thanked the Lord for now she had "come to a place where I can have a comfortable home for the rest of my days." Another woman arrived at the asylum after being found living "a lonely and solitary life by the lake shore." Similarly, sixty-year-old Mary had no home and was jailed after she was found wandering around town occupying deserted buildings. In a more premeditated manner, Patrick Maloney, aged sixty-one and "broken down by poverty and want," admitted to having burnt down a barn. Despite doubts as to whether he had actually performed the crime, he was placed in jail and later in the Rockwood Asylum. Once secure there, he stated that he had confessed to the crime to ensure that he would be imprisoned and have a home.

A complete lack of family was a more frequent cause of committal than having been abandoned by relatives. While less than 10 per cent of the overall population remained single in nineteenth-century Ontario, over 16 per cent of Rockwood's elderly patients were single.[31] Another 26 per cent of those admitted were widowed. This figure was also higher than the portion of widowed old people in the general population. Roughly half of the old people in Rockwood had a living spouse, but married people formed a considerably higher portion

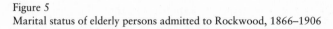

Figure 5
Marital status of elderly persons admitted to Rockwood, 1866–1906

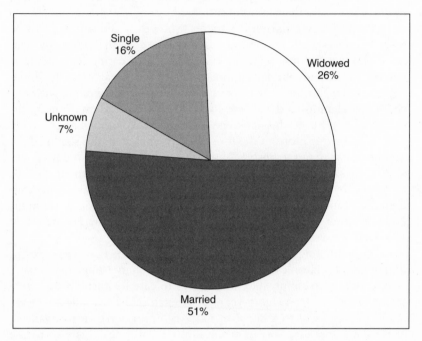

(75 per cent) of the general population outside the asylum. Among the aged alone, roughly two-thirds of the total population was married. (See Figure 5.)

People with no living children also formed a greater portion of the population inside the asylum than they did outside its walls. Although one-quarter of the case files do not indicate how many children a patient had, over 30 per cent of the patients for whom the number of children was reported had none. In a further 8 per cent of these cases the individual had only one child. Of the aged people admitted to the institution during the nineteenth century, 134 or 43 per cent of them had previously been cared for by a family member. Almost three-quarters of these people had been cared for by a spouse or a child, mainly wives and daughters. (See Figure 6.) Although siblings, nieces, nephews, and even neighbours took care of single or childless people, in most cases the absence of immediate family members meant that an aged person had no one to look after them when they became incapable of doing so for themselves. The patients of Rockwood bear testimony to the fact that having no relatives at hand to provide care greatly increased an old person's chances of being placed in an asylum.

Figure 6
Persons caring for the aged before their admission to Rockwood[32]

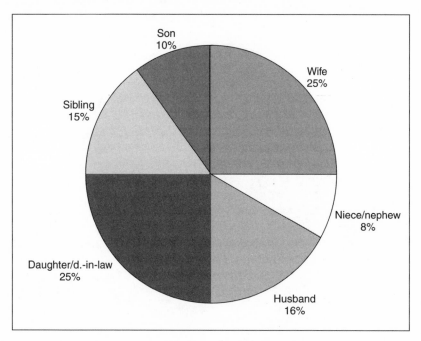

Of those people who were not cared for by their families before being admitted to Rockwood, the bulk, excepting those transferred from other asylums, were sent there from houses of industry, houses of providence or refuge, and hospitals. These charitable institutions for the poor were the only other facilities that dealt with the aged and destitute. Such institutions, however, refused to retain individuals who required extra attention or those who had become unmanageable. Although government policy intended that old people suffering from mild mental decay be cared for in houses of industry, this was not often possible since the other residents complained about being disturbed by the "gibbering idiots."[33] It was certainly common in England for workhouses and local administrators to send the people who were the most troublesome and expensive to maintain to the asylum.[34] Similarly, both the Kingston House of Industry and the House of Providence frequently sent aged people to the Rockwood Asylum once their behaviour exceeded what those institutions considered proper.[35] Once the House of Industry ejected someone, the insane asylum was the last resort. The patients who did not arrive at Rockwood from one of these institutions were, for the most part, on their own before their admis-

Figure 7
Origins of aged patients who did not live with their families

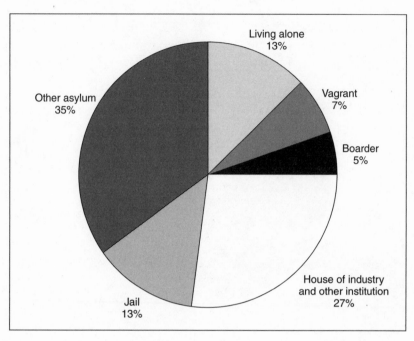

sion. Over 10 per cent lived alone, 7 per cent were homeless vagrants, and 5 per cent were boarders. (See Figure 7.) These figures show that, rather than being negligent towards their ill and aged relatives, or being eager to abandon them to the "tender care of the community," families, especially spouses and children, played a crucial role in providing care that kept many elderly out of institutions.

Historians such as Gerald Grob and John Walton claim that, instead of being institutionalized because their families could not be bothered to care for them, those aged people who did have relatives were usually committed to asylums because their kin lacked the resources necessary to maintain them and they had no other options.[36] As well, Walton confirms that, rather than being merely inconvenient, people who were sent to asylums were usually violent, disruptive, and difficult to handle.[37]

People may have been willing to assist their kin but this did not mean that they were able to do so. The burdens of even minimal nursing care were frequently beyond the resources of nineteenth-century families.[38] Providing physical care for an elderly person, especially when mental illness or senility made them difficult to manage, was usually an arduous task. Some people were simply too ill or feeble themselves to undertake the care of another. For instance, one man explained in a letter that he could not care for his wife since he was poor, ill, and in need of medical attention himself. Sometimes, too, people who were willing to look after an aged relative often found that they had conflicting responsibilities to other people, usually their spouses, children, or employers.[39]

Even when a person was potentially manageable at home, some families did not have the resources to cope with the financial burden. Almost all Rockwood's patients came from poor families. As one observer commented in 1885, "Rockwood's five hundred and five residents were paupers, with the exception of the very few who pay the cost of their own maintenance."[40] People from poor families could simply not afford to halt their daily activities, especially the work that provided their livelihood, to remain by an elderly person's side. One woman, for example, could not remain at home because she could not be left alone. Her presence prevented her husband from going to work, which was something he had to do to survive. It is understandable that most people did not have the energy or the time both to earn a living and to care for a family member. When the asylum officials requested that one women remove her father from the asylum because he "was well enough to be cared for at home," she lamented that "I cannot do for my father as I should like to. I work long hours to keep a roof over my head and food to eat. I have no means whatever to pay for an attendant on my father. I dare not stop work to wait upon him, even if I was strong enough to do it." As the care required by an ill older person increased and began to demand more and more of a relative's, or even an entire family's, time and energy, these compounded obligations often became more than many individuals or families could handle.[41]

Once a family had reached the limits of their power to care for someone, there were few places they could go for help.[42] In Ontario, official attitudes towards assisting families who were caring for the ill and insane hardened noticeably in the latter decades of the century. In 1857 the superintendent of the Toronto Asylum for the Insane had acknowledged that there were in the asylum several senile old people "who with adequate legislative provision for their support may live locally" and might have been "permitted the continuance of the most prized of all human privileges, personal liberty."[43] By the end of the century, in contrast, it was felt that, while assistance could be provided to individuals caring for unrelated people, "it would be unwise to pay relatives for the care of their own."[44] Hence, there was little assistance or relief available for families caring for the senile. While families may have been willing to care for their kin, with no form of financial assistance available to people attempting to cope with the "considerable demands"[45] of caregiving, they had no choice but to institutionalize their dependent elderly relatives or face financial ruin.[46] Others were forced to send their kin away to protect themselves from emotional trauma or actual bodily harm. It is easy to judge families harshly, by modern standards, for providing inadequate care or for relinquishing their caring functions, but in the atmosphere of the late nineteenth century many families may not have had other alternatives if the family was to survive.[47] In this regard, nineteenth-century families came to view institutions "as regrettable but indispensable necessities."[48]

Finding an institution that was willing to care for an aged person who required special care was difficult. As mentioned previously, most institutions such as houses of industry and refuge refused to admit or retain aged people who were not able to conform to those institutions' expectations of proper behaviour.[49] Often, insane asylums were the only place a family could send a senile or difficult-to-manage older person. For these reasons, desperate families frequently had to resort to what could easily be interpreted as a form of "granny-dumping" or abandonment by placing their physically, emotionally, and mentally ill elderly people in insane asylums. Regardless of the problems associated with sending the aged to mental asylums, this course of action was often forced upon families by public policies that left them no alternative but to utilize the limited resources the government made available to them. Whether they were adequate or not, insane asylums were the only places a confused or ill aged person could receive anywhere near the amount of supervision or medical care they needed.[50]

From the moment a family sought to commit an ill relative to an asylum, their actions were regulated by government polices which forced families to treat their kin in a less than exemplary fashion. Regulations dictated that there were two methods by which a family could have a difficult-to-manage person admitted into an insane asylum: ordinary process and warrants. Families seeking to admit a relative through ordinary process needed three physicians to certify that the person was insane. After a person had been certified, he or she would be eligible for admission into a hospital once a bed became available. Given the crowded state of the province's asylums during most of the nineteenth century, it was almost impossible for a person to gain admission to an asylum in this way. People could wait for months and still see no vacancy appear.[51]

Warrants were a more expedient process. Public authorities such as justices of the peace, magistrates, or jail doctors could confine someone in a local jail and then issue a warrant testifying that this individual was a "dangerous lunatic" meaning that he posed a threat to himself or the community. Asylums were forced to admit warrant patients regardless of the number of free beds. Hence, many families found themselves forced to have their kin imprisoned and declared insane and dangerous in order to secure their admission to an asylum.[52] As the medical superintendent of the Rockwood asylum declared in 1882: "Many patients sought admission through ordinary process, but owing to the crowded state of the asylum and our inability to receive them, promptly many of these applicants were afterwards committed to a jail and transferred to the asylum under warrant."[53] Under such a system it was almost impossible for a family to send their relatives to an asylum in a humane manner. Thus, aside from the basic stigma attached to being treated for mental illness,[54] the "indignity" of being committed to a nineteenth-century asylum often included being confined in one of the province's "squalid and inhumane" district jails.[55] Almost one-third of the elderly people in Rockwood arrived there from a cell in a county jail after having been labelled "dangerous lunatics." Many people were designated as "dangerous" merely because that was what was necessary to get them into the asylum.

Rockwood's chief medical superintendent remarked in 1899 that the fact so many patients "should have had to pass through the gaols before reaching this institution is a reproach to the people of the district from which we receive admissions."[56] What the superintendent failed to mention in this indictment of the populace was that, once someone became unmanageable at home, a family often had no choice but to send that person to a jail since this was the only way to ensure that he would eventually be sent to an asylum where he could, it was hoped, be properly cared for. Despite decades of protest from various doctors and magistrates, the government did little to modify the policy that forced families into their predicament.

Asylum officials complained that many families used the warrants as a means of abandoning helpless old people for whom they no longer wished to care. They claimed that aged people, being merely "in their dotage," posed no threat to society and could, in most cases, be "easily cared for at home."[57] While it may have been true that most of these difficult-to-manage elderly people were suffering from the ravages of senile dementia and were not actually insane, this did not mean that they could be easily looked after by their families. Senile old people regularly demanded far more care than most families could sustain either physically or financially. Some gerontologists have argued that the term senile is merely "a medical expression of despair applied to socially isolated old people for whom nobody will accept responsibility."[58] In most instances, however, the Rockwood asylum patients described as senile were truly ill and suffering from a disease that caused "a complete disruption of the personality," the result of which was that "eventually nothing of the patient's former personality [was] recognizable."[59] Often, symptoms of paranoia, especially delusions of persecution and unrealistic jealousies, caused a person to become unpredictable, violent, abusive, and dangerous.[60] These, indeed, were the reasons the vast majority of the aged people in the Rockwood asylum were sent there. Almost all the aged people admitted to the institution between 1858 and 1906 were described as "uncontrollable," "violent to themselves or others," or "suicidal." Many were all three.[61] (See Figure 8.)

These designations were likely, in some cases, exaggerations of the patient's actual condition. Yet the fact that families and local officials sometimes lied about the actual "danger" certain aged people posed to society does not mean that they were not concerned about their well-being. It merely indicates that families did what was necessary in order to conform to government policies and ensure that their aged kin received what was often the only form of care available to them. The overall impression that emerges from these case files is that, rather than resorting to institutionalization at the first possible opportunity, nineteenth-century families used public institutions only as a desperate last resort.[62]

This was especially true when violence was involved. As the medical superintendent remarked in 1879, "patients are retained at home as long as they can be managed by the members of the household, they are at last sent to the asylum when they have become violent."[63] Also, even when a person's violent or uncontrollable behaviour was exaggerated and that individual did not pose a danger to society, a family could have difficulty coping with the actual degree of violence or unmanageability being exhibited. In certain cases, for instance, an uncontrollable person was one who required constant watching. The care of such a person, aside from taking time and energy which many people did not have to spare, could be emotionally taxing, frustrating, and disruptive to an entire family. Families were regularly forced to commit their aged kin to an asylum to preserve not only their financial security but also their emotional and even their physical well-being. Several people, for example, were prone to wandering out of their homes and disappearing, putting themselves in danger, frightening their families, and upsetting their neighbours. Ann, aged seventy-five, would wander five or six kilometres before her family could find her. She had to be watched constantly to keep her from breaking the furniture or harming herself – she was fond of standing in front of trains. Her son and neighbours finally could not cope any longer and committed her in 1888.

Other patients posed greater problems. Jonathan, admitted to Rockwood in 1897, tore down his daughter's stove pipes, turned on the gas, and tossed her clothing out the window. Thomas was even more de-

Figure 8
Proportion of aged persons admitted to Rockwood as violent, dangerous, or suicidal

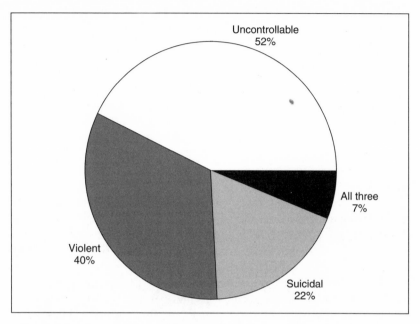

structive, breaking doors and windows, tearing down fences, and rip-ping up clothing. Yet another man, aged eighty, repeatedly tried to burn down his home with his family in it. Ellen, meanwhile, was sent to the asylum after her actions threatened to ruin her son financially; she had killed his geese and damaged his apple trees. Numerous aged people became suicidal and could not be kept at home because the moment they were not watched they would attempt to kill themselves. Many families simply could not provide the degree of surveillance necessary to prevent a tragedy. One daughter said of her mother that "it was im-possible to do anything with her": on separate occasions she had tried to hang herself, poison herself, and drown herself. These suicidal peo-ple were often quite persistent and could become violent when their families tried to deter them from their purpose.

While most Victorians refused to consider suicide acceptable, many suicidal patients felt that they had valid reasons for ending their lives. One woman wanted her throat cut because she had gone blind. Others feared being destitute and alone and believed that "they might as well go to Hell sooner than later." Still others were simply "tired of living." They were committed to Rockwood, not only because it was assumed that anyone who tried to end their life was insane, but also because families felt that it was the only way to prevent their loved one from achieving their goal. Regardless of the precautions taken, some patients succeeded in ending their lives, even after being committed to the asylum. One woman hung herself with her bedsheets, another patient jumped out a window, and a third drowned himself. Still others simply refused to eat and, though they were usually forced-fed, most died after a short time.

More than being a nuisance, certain senile old people were institutionalized because they had become a genuine threat to the safety and well-being of their families. While officials did sometimes exaggerate the degree to which aged people were violent or dangerous, the description did fit numerous patients. The asylum doctors recognized that these individuals had become violent and abusive, particularly to the very people who were doing the most to care for them. This was the case with sixty-year-old Mary. Her husband tried to manage her for two years until she became so violent that he found that he could not sleep for fear his wife would kill him. Asylum officials reported that she was deceitful and vicious and hurt other patients. Similarly, seventy-year-old Catherine suddenly took a strong dislike to the daughter who had been caring for her. She became increasingly threatening, and eventually the daughter was forced to commit her mother after she had attempted to harm her with a knife. In another instance, John began chasing his wife with a knife and driving her out of the house. After a short time she became too terrified of her husband to keep him at home.

Other people such as Barbara became a menace to her entire family. The seventy-six-year-old threw lighted lamps at her daughter and tried to knock her down the stairs. She hit her grandchildren, threw dishes at them, and finally tried to burn down the entire house. Another woman, eighty years old, threatened her grandchildren with a knife and could never be left alone with children for fear she might kill them. One man began to drag his invalid daughter about by her hair, while another would lock his family in a room and try to sell the house, with them in it.

Violent and unpredictable aged people were not only impossible to care for but the emotional trauma caused by their actions provoked serious rifts among other family members. One man was said to be "highly disturbing to all members of his family." His "familial home unit has been destroyed by his threatening mood." Gerald Grob explains that "the internal disruption of the family that followed certain forms of behaviour ultimately reached a crisis stage." Once this occurred the "decision to commit the person causing the crisis rested on the belief that the welfare of the family as a whole had to take precedence."[64]

In other cases, the frustration, anger, and sheer exhaustion brought on by caring for a difficult-to-manage person could have even more tragic consequences.[65] Although we will never know the full extent of elder abuse in the past, the records of Rockwood Asylum indicate that in some cases the aged were treated violently by their caregivers. Eighty-year-old Rose arrived at Rockwood after having been "thrown forcibly against a pile of cord-wood." Daniel was admitted "terribly bruised and cut about the face, a gash existed over each eye and the nose was cut." The asylum reported that "this man has evidently been badly taken care of at home. He seems to bear the marks of direct violence." One woman told all the neighbours that her sister "pounds her," while others were simply, "badly treated by ... family." In such cases, old people were better off in an institution than they were at home. [66]

While some family members were truly abusive people, in several instances elder abuse was likely the result of a family member being expected to provide far more care than he or she was capable of. Also, in moments of frustration, the violence inflicted by family members upon the aged could have been a reaction to the abuse senile persons inflicted upon their caregivers. It is also probable that, had there been some form of assistance available to these families sooner, the abuse may not have occurred.

Even when a family was willing to keep an unmanageable relative at home, this often became impossible once the person began to disturb their neighbours. As Cheryl Warsh explains, middle-class Victorians felt that families had a responsibility towards the community to control potentially bothersome kin. Disturbed individuals were not only a "cause of grief to their friends," they created "uneasiness and alarm" in the community.[67] If a family could no longer prevent a confused older person from becoming a nuisance to the neighbours they were often obliged to remove the offending person to a place where they would not cause such problems.[68]

In several instances, the case files of elderly patients stress that they were sent for psychiatric care largely because their behaviour had become intolerable to their neighbours and community. William, for instance, a once unobtrusive man, was committed in 1896 after he became a nuisance to his community; he was disturbing businesses by threatening lawsuits for no reason. A Napanee man arrived at Rockwood after the community complained that he hung around and "disturbed the ladies and chased young children." One woman was described as "plaguing the neighbours" because she wandered into strangers' homes at all hours and destroyed their property. Yet another patient was committed in 1891 after reports that he had terrified his neighbours by firing a gun at them. In an even more dramatic example, sixty-five-year-old Charles was described as "a terror to the ladies of Belleville" because he "exceeded the bounds of propriety" and chased about the streets any handsome young woman. Another patient was a "source of great disturbance to her neighbourhood." The seventy-six-year-old woman ran from one home to another seeking protection from imaginary dangers. All these patients became more than just a concern to their families; they were obviously disrupting the daily lives of their entire community. At this point their families had little choice but to commit them.

In spite of the odds against keeping a senile relative at home, the Rockwood case files indicate that relatives regularly provided care for as long as they could, even once an aged person became demented and difficult to deal with. Letters to the administrators of the asylum from the families of patients confirm that many families made every attempt to retain their elderly relatives at home as long as possible and gave up their kin out of necessity, not choice. Seventy-eight year-old Rebecca had been placed in the Hastings county jail in 1890 when she became violent and uncontrollable. Rather than have her sent to an asylum, her daughter and son-in-law requested that she be released into their custody. Eventually, however, they, too, found her impossible to control and were forced to send her to Rockwood. One daughter had been her father's "constant attendant," but he was suicidal and had "put her through much distress" until she finally was forced to abandon her attempts to care for him at home. Eighty-year-old Mary became unmanageable. But, when one relative could not care for her any longer, she was sent to another. It was not until her entire family finally discovered that "no one can manage her" that she was sent to Rockwood.

Even after placing a relative in Rockwood, most families did not give up on them entirely or abandon them. Some families, changing their minds out of guilt or merely because they had had a month or two of rest, insisted that their kin be returned to them, occasionally against the advice of the asylum doctors. Several patients were discharged "unimproved" at the request of their kin. For example, Frederick was admitted to Rockwood in January 1889 as uncontrollable and suicidal. By May his family had decided that they wanted to care for him and took him home although "the doctors do not consider it a good idea." Another woman was warned that her father would require constant care and that "unless someone is prepared to devote most of their time to looking after him" it would be best to "leave him here." Some patients, such as William or sixty-nine-year-old Mary, were taken back by their families only to be returned a few months later when once again their families found them too difficult to manage. Other families took their

kin out on two- and three-month probation periods. Still other families, knowing they were unable to care for their kin, insisted that their
relative be returned to them once they heard that the patient was dying
since, even if he could not be cared for at home, they did not wish him
to "die in the asylum."

All these cases offer proof that families did not abandon the aged in
asylums. They used the asylum to help them cope with the terrible
problem of providing care for family members for whom they themselves could not care. Sometimes caregivers only needed a short respite
before they felt able to resume their duties; others relied on the asylum
but provided periodic care. Some families could only visit their kin, and
some eventually stopped doing so. Often, however, this was due not to
the family's lack of willingness but to the fact that asylum administrators made family members feel unwelcome since they did not appreciate or encourage family intervention in patient care.[69] While families
were willing to assist asylum doctors care for their relatives, asylum officials were rarely willing to do the same for families.

In some cases the asylum doctors insisted on releasing individuals to
the care of their family, especially if the patient was aged and considered simply a chronic case, even though the family insisted that they
could not handle the person. The asylum officials would argue that patient was "quiet and harmless" and did not need asylum care; the family, however, would assert that at home the patient was unmanageable.
John Walton reports that this practice was common in England, where
asylum officials tried to release quieter patients to workhouses or to the
care of their families. Many of these patients "lost their tranquillity"
and had to be returned.[70] In Rockwood, William was one such case.
He was admitted and discharged as "improved" several times only to
be returned to the asylum a few months later by his family who insisted
that he was not well. One explanation for this pattern is that some senile persons, having taken a dislike to a particular individual, would
become deranged only in the presence of that individual. Once away
from their spouse or child or other family member, these people would
become calm. It does not seem, however, that asylum officials were
willing to accept that some people behaved differently around their
family than they did around strangers. By releasing patients into the
care of the very person or persons who caused them to become upset
and frequently violent, officials caused a great deal of grief for both the
patients and the hapless family member that had to deal with them.

That people were committed to Rockwood as a last resort and that
they were committed for justifiable reasons does not mean that the
asylum was necessarily a humane or safe place for the elderly. While
families hoped that asylums would prove helpful to their troubled or

senile relatives, many old, feeble patients in these institutions became
victims of younger violent residents.[71] One such dangerous person, it
was reported, would "exercise his bloodthirsty propensities whenever
the opportunity arises, upon our helpless and inoffensive inmates; and
it is noteworthy that he selects for his victims those who are unable to
offer much if any resistance."[72] Among the helpless victims of these
violent residents was Felix, a man over seventy, who was attacked and
beaten by the patients sleeping in his dormitory. He was left un-
conscious and died a few days later. Another old man was knocked
down and accidentally killed in 1868. Serious injuries were more common. For instance, in 1885 Mary, "an old woman in wretched health,"
was "knocked about and kicked black and blue." Another patient,
Anne, was attacked with a chair in 1885 and struck with a boot a year
later.

Aged patients themselves were responsible for some of this violence.
Martha was notorious for attacking, scratching, and "pounding" other
patients, most of them elderly. Similarly, Sarah was known for "committing assault often." In 1886 these two patients fought each other,
Sarah ending up with a dislocated hip. Sixty-five-year-old John was imprisoned and then sent to Rockwood for assaulting his wife and others.
Once in the institution he continued in his violent ways, often assaulting other patients. There was also sixty-year-old Norah, who was "always ready to do a little prize fighting." Of course, since most patients
were committed to Rockwood because they were violent, dangerous,
or unmanageable, it is not surprising that the asylum was a violent and
dangerous place. The instances of violent aged people confirm that not
every warrant describing an old person as "dangerous" was inaccurate.

Because senile elderly patients were considered chronic and incurable, they were often shuttled from one asylum to another in order to
make room for more treatable cases. These transfers uprooted confused old people from their familiar environment and placed them in
strange surroundings far away from their old home. In some cases, old
people were transferred not once, but two, three, and four times. It is
doubtful that such peregrinations could have done much to improve
the mental state of the patients concerned. Lydia, for instance, arrived
at Rockwood in 1878 at the age of seventy-five. She was transferred to
the Toronto asylum in 1889 when she was eighty-six years old. Similarly, Hugh began his asylum residence in London at the age of sixty-
one. After five years he was transferred to the Toronto asylum, where
he stayed for only six months before being sent to Rockwood in 1885.
From there he was sent to the Hamilton asylum in 1888. In another example of a person who was moved about the province for little apparent reason, sixty-five-year-old Joseph was jailed in 1884 and sent to

Rockwood. Six years later he was transferred to Toronto and then in 1895 he was returned to Rockwood, where he died shortly thereafter.

Many modern-day commentators have condemned nineteenth-century families for allowing their aged relatives to be exposed to the horrors of insane asylums. Yet the records of one such institution, the Rockwood asylum, demonstrate that this criticism is unfair. Senile old people required not only extraordinary amounts of care but care of a specialized nature that was well beyond the means of most nineteenth-century families and indeed remains beyond the capabilities of most families today. Further, the fact that asylums were the only place the senile aged could be sent was not the fault of families. Neither was the manner in which the senile were admitted to these institutions. Families merely made use of the limited resources supplied to them by government, and followed the rules and procedures dictated to them by various government policies, to obtain whatever care they could for their needy kin as well as to save themselves from what could amount to a life of "continual danger, dreadful anxiety, and the necessity of constant watching."[73] They can hardly be blamed if the care in asylums was inadequate, inhuman, or insufficient. The blame rather rests with government.

It was public policies, not a lack of concern for the aged, that caused nineteenth-century families to subject their aged members to the unpleasant environment of mental institutions. The asylum was a final resource for desperate families rather than an easy option for the uncaring or irresponsible.[74]

CHAPTER SEVEN

Long-Term-Care Reform and Family Obligations in Ontario in the 1990s

It is clear that nineteenth-century institutional or long-term-care policies had a negative impact on the aged, who found it difficult to receive the care they required, and on their families, who had to shoulder the burden of caring for those aged people who were deemed ineligible for institutional care. What is unclear, however, is whether the government policies that created these problems for the aged and their families actually benefitted the state in any way.

Despite reducing social spending in relation to all other government spending, enforcing family obligations for caregiving, and restricting the elderly's access to institutional care, the demand for long-term care for aged people continued to increase. By 1903 the government was forced to make the construction of county houses of refuge or industry mandatory in response to a sharp rise in the numbers of people needing institutional care, many of them elderly.[1] Yet it also continued to restrict its responsibility for the aged by making the family primarily responsible for their care.

In 1921 the Ontario government passed the Parents' Maintenance Act, which allowed magistrates to order children to make weekly support payments to their dependent elderly parents. Once again the legislature ignored the fact that the children of most destitute older people were also living in poverty.[2] Rather than admit the true nature and extent of the problem, it was easier to argue that families were merely irresponsible. As with most measures aimed at reducing the state's financial responsibilities towards the dependent aged by passing them on to the later-born, the Parents' Maintenance Act did little to solve the problems of the aged or the state. A completely ineffectual piece of legislation which was seldom enforced,[3] it failed to alleviate the financial, emotional, and physical suffering of either the aged or their families which the emphasis on family obligations had helped create.

Ann Shola Orloff argues that the much publicized poverty of the aged at the turn-of-the century was, in fact, not a natural element of old age or the result of the irresponsibility of families. It was instead a direct result of government policies which restricted the access of the aged to the care they required and placed upon their families burdens of care with which they were entirely unable to cope.[4] In this sense, the enforcement of family obligations backfired, as a cost-saving measure, since it was the poverty and suffering created by such policies that led older and younger people alike to fight for the implementation of old age pensions for the aged poor.

Pensions, it was argued, would prevent some aged people from becoming financially dependent while allowing others who did become physically dependent to contribute towards their own care, thus relieving their families of part of the burden they were carrying. Orloff suggests, therefore, that demands for new forms of public assistance for the aged, which became especially strong in the early part of this century, were directly tied to the reductions in spending on services for the dependent aged initiated by late-nineteenth-century governments in Canada, Great Britain, and the United States.[5]

The Canadian government eventually did implement means-tested old age pensions for the dependent elderly, the costs of which were shared by the federal government, the provinces and, in Ontario, the municipalities.[6] These pensions provided a certain amount of relief for some financially dependent older people; however, they did little for those in need of more than just financial assistance. The Ontario government did not improve to any significant extent either the quality or the availability of institutional or long-term care for the physically or mentally dependent elderly.

Despite the periodic and rapid expansion of public residential facilities, the government has never been able to provide anywhere near the number of beds required to accommodate all the people who require care.[7] For example, while the population of Toronto grew by 500 per cent between 1900 and 1940, institutional accommodation for the elderly only doubled.[8] James Struthers describes how in post-war Ontario this lack of government-funded accommodation led to the development of a substantial and largely unregulated private nursing-home industry. By 1957 the problems associated with a lack of public accommodation for the elderly and the proliferation of unsupervised private-care facilities inspired the first conference on aging at the University of Toronto to recognize that there was an "emerging crisis in long-term care."[9]

By 1958 the province had begun to deal with the problem by subsidizing and at least partially regulating private nursing homes. Yet the government did not substantially increase the number of beds available in provincial institutions. Further, because it continued to emphasize institutional care, few alternatives to such care were developed. In these circumstances, the shortage of public institutional facilities meant that many people who required care but who were unable to afford a private nursing home were forced to survive without the services they needed. The problem was not alleviated until 1972, when nursing-home care was declared eligible for coverage under the Ontario Hospital Insurance Plan. Since 1945, then, the overall result of the growing need for institutional care combined with the lack of public accommodation was that, when it came to the care of the dependent elderly, the provincial government relied increasingly upon private institutions. In fact, by 1986, 86 per cent of the long-term-care beds in Ontario were located in private nursing homes.[10]

By the late 1970s even the combined resources of the private nursing-home sector and the provincial homes for the aged were unable to meet the demand for institutional care in the province. It was reported in 1977 that there was "a crying need" for appropriate accomodation for senior citizens.[11] With chronic-care hospitals filled to capacity and long waiting lists for nursing homes, acute-care hospitals and homes for the aged dominated legislative discussions about the elderly during most of the 1980s.[12] A situation similar to the nineteenth century had developed, in which the government's focus on institutional care was producing an ever growing demand for services. Besides failing to develop alternatives, government refused to expand institutional facilities to meet the need that had been at least partially created by its own policies. By 1992, 4,300 Ontarians were said to be waiting for long-term residential care. In the meantime, most were being cared for by their families.[13]

Not surprisingly, predictions of even larger increases in the number of older people needing care in the future have caused the government to see the problem as a crisis. Yet, despite the enormous changes that have occurred in the economy, in the political structure, and in society in general since the 1890s, the basic approach of governments to the challenge of providing care for the dependent aged has remained the same. Recent policies are certainly far more subtle, sophisticated, and complex than earlier ones, and the details of the debates have also changed dramatically. What is similar, however, is the overall emphasis on reducing the state's responsibility for the dependent aged by limiting the provision of institutional care, thereby transferring a greater degree of responsibility onto the community and ultimately the family. Even the explanations given for such actions are similar in that recent governments have, like their nineteenth-century counterparts, utilized no-

Figure 9
Increase in the elderly population of Ontario compared to the total population,
1983–2001

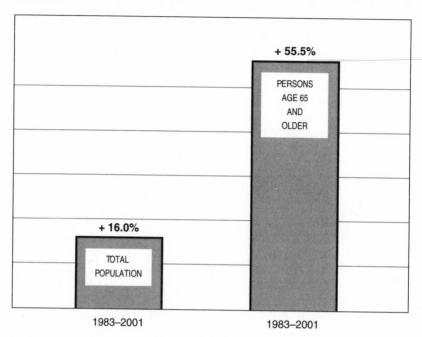

tions of population aging, old-age dependency, and family obligations
to justify policies of fiscal restraint. Although what follows is only a
cursory examination of these trends, it suggests that there are sufficient
similarities between current policies and nineteenth-century ones to
raise questions about the apparent direction of current long-term-care
policies and the impact they may have on the aged, their families, and
the state.

POPULATION AGING

As in the final decades of the nineteenth century, population aging has
dominated recent discussions about the provision of services to the dependent elderly. During the last decade in particular, population aging
has been highlighted as a major problem by MPPs of all parties. In
1992, during the debates over Bill 101, An Act to Amend Previous Acts
Concerning Long-Term Care (namely the Charitable Institutions Act,
the Homes for the Aged Act, and the Nursing Homes Act), Conservative, Liberal and NDP members of the legislature presented or com-

mented on various statistics revealing the extent of population aging in Ontario.[14] *A New Agenda*, the Liberal Party's 1986 policy statement on long-term care, included a particularly alarming graph highlighting the expected growth in the size of the aged population. The impact of the graph was made all the more dramatic by a comparison of the size of the aged population to the total population. The overall impression given was that by 2001 the aged will actually outnumber the non-aged.[15] (See Figure 9.)

To Ontario legislators over the last decade, population aging presented "some unique problems"[16] and was a definite cause for concern. As NDP member David Warner warned, "we are getting a larger and larger elderly population and we're not ready for it."[17] Throughout the legislative debates of the period, population aging was characterized as a potential crisis, especially in health care, where the aged will in the future "place an unprecedented pressure"[18] or "increasingly heavy demands on an already overburdened system."[19] Liberal MPP Margaret Campbell claimed that "older people, by their very nature will be calling on the health delivery system."[20] Even the minister of seniors affairs, Ron Van Horne, reported in 1986 that "there is no question that the utilization of health and social services increases with age, yet, most people do not fully appreciate the magnitude of this trend and its implications for our society and government."[21]

OLD-AGE DEPENDENCY

In recent years, as in the last century, the perception of population aging as a social problem has been closely related to the image of the aged as a largely dependent group. Conservative Bruce McCaffery reported in 1980 that, among "all of us in politics," there was "a tendency to think that after one has celebrated one's 65th birthday one is then quickly approaching a point where one becomes the responsibility of the state and that people in this category are unwilling or unable to provide for themselves."[22] Other MPPs similarly highlighted the poverty and dependence of the aged. Marion Bryden of the NDP noted in the legislature that "we know many of them [the aged] live below the poverty line,"[23] and Liberal Margaret Campbell claimed that the elderly often seem to be "divorced from their family, isolated and lonely."[24] A "Current Issues Paper," intended as background information for legislators, stated that "poverty provides the essential context for the lives of many elderly people."[25] Such images of the aged as a growing population of poor, lonely, and ill people played a large role in determining the scope and direction of long-term care reforms in a period of economic crisis and fiscal restraint.

FISCAL RESTRAINT

During the Liberal administration of David Peterson (1985–90), the standing committee on social development indicated that, in 1988, 14 per cent of the annual provincial budget, or $5 billion, was spent on services for the 11 per cent of the population represented by Ontario's more than 1 million aged people. Addressing the predicted costs associated with population aging, the committee stated that while the government must ensure that appropriate services were available to the elderly, it must also be fiscally responsible.[26] Even NDP members quoted Senator David Croll when he pointed out that the funds for maintaining the elderly in the future would not materialize out of thin air; the money would have to come either from savings in this generation or from taxes in following generations.[27]

Since 1988, as the overall economic situation in Ontario has worsened and concern over the deficit has dominated policy discussions, fiscal restraint has become the central principal of most government policy, especially in the realm of social spending.[28] As in the nineteenth century, when it came to social spending on the elderly in particular, the government has focused on reducing the cost of long-term institutional care and devising cheaper alternatives at the community level.

INSTITUTIONAL CARE
FOR THE DEPENDENT AGED

Debates over long-term care have emphasized that institutionalization is the most expensive form of care. For example, government reports have highlighted the fact that, once inside institutions, some seniors were provided with expensive and often unnecessary medical treatments while others were over-drugged. In 1986 alone it was discovered that these treatments wasted about $855 million in Ontario.[29] Instead of focusing upon eliminating such abuses, however, the government used this evidence to promote policies of de-institutionalization. From the late 1980s, the focus of long-term-care reform became limiting institutional care and replacing it with community-based programs. Although community care, in its ideal form, would be an improvement over institutionalization for many seniors, the type of community care envisioned by recent government policies – driven as they have been mainly by the goal of fiscal restraint – would likely leave much to be desired. Community care has been promoted largely because, being "all done by volunteers,"[30] it is assumed to be less expensive.

As well as assuming that community care was less expensive than institutional care, legislators claimed that "too many seniors are institutionalized needlessly."[31] This assertion permitted the government to argue that there was no need to construct new facilities or expand existing ones because the existing system of residential-care facilities already had sufficient space to accommodate the people who "really should be there." As in the 1890s, the government argued that its job was to remove from institutions, or restrict the access to institutions, of all those people who did not belong there. It was assumed that all the people who were defined as not really needing institutional care could be adequately cared for by community-based services.[32] This assumption certainly helped the government justify the closing of twenty nursing homes in 1992.[33]

The Ontario Nursing Home Association (ONHA), however, challenged the government's reasoning. In its 1992 report on long-term-care reform, the association pointed out that a survey of nursing-home residents revealed that between 60 and 80 per cent of them were cognitively impaired and that a large portion were disturbed and difficult to manage owing to such traits as aggression, depression, wandering, resistance to care, sexually inappropriate conduct, and hallucinations. Further, 76 per cent of nursing-home residents required assistance when eating, 70 per cent were incontinent, and 60 per cent experienced difficulty communicating.[34] The association contended that, rather than being institutionalized needlessly, the bulk of their residents could not be cared for adequately within the community. It also demonstrated that one was far more likely to find seniors in the community who needed institutional care but who could not access it than to locate elderly people who had been institutionalized needlessly.[35]

Nevertheless, the government continued to reduce or freeze funding for institutional care and limit the construction of new institutions. The ONHA argued that the result of these decisions would be that, as the number of old people increased over the coming decades, the ratio of institutional beds to the aged population would decrease significantly. In other words, community care, rather then being an option, would become an absolute necessity for a large segment of the dependent aged population simply because few seniors would be able to enter an institution regardless of the type of care they required.[36]

For reasons such as these, the combination of a move towards community care for the aged with a concern for fiscal restraint has made many people sceptical about the ultimate goals and fearful of the overall impact of long-term-care reforms. For example, the NDP government of Bob Rae (1990–95) was criticized because, although it was eager to save money by reducing spending on institutions and initiating cuts to the number of chronic-care beds, in funding for homes for the aged, and in the number of nursing-home beds, it seemed less anxious to ensure that sufficient new funding was provided to ensure that an adequate support network was available in the community to care for all those people who would no longer be able to access institutional accommodation.[37] It was reported that hospital services were being curtailed at a time when funding for local home-support programs was being reduced across the province.[38] As well, some voiced the concern that planned hospital restructuring would result in fewer beds being made available to the aged and that elderly patients would be expelled from hospitals sooner on the assumption that community-care services would be able to provide the care that hospitals would no longer provide. In other words, it appeared that the government was using home-care/community-care rhetoric to justify drastically reducing the size of Ontario's institutional-care system.

FAMILIES AND LONG-TERM CARE-REFORM

The fiscal-restraint elements of long-term-care reform are of particular significance to the families of aged people. Despite the histrionics about the need for the government to provide adequate services for the aged within the community, it appears that in their practical application recent suggestions concerning the reform of long-term care contain the potential to put into place a major redistribution of responsibilities between the state and the family regarding the care of the dependent aged.

Just as an increase in community-care programs is supposed to be a necessary element of policies aimed at the de-institutionalization of the aged, it appears that an increase in amount of care families provide for the aged is a necessary, if unspoken, element of community-care programs. Over the last decade, all three political parties assumed that families would play a key role in the transfer of services for the dependent aged from institutions to the community. In this sense, politicians were well aware that long-term-care reform involved a discussion about the boundaries between state responsibilities and family obligations. To the Liberal government, one of the key questions concerning the care of the aged was "how to determine where families should be doing something for their parents, where the government should be doing it for their parents and where it ends."[39]

As well, when it came to determining where the boundary between state responsibilities and families obligations should be, all three parties made it clear that they expected families to do more. A key assumption surrounding the implementation of community-care policies is that caring for dependent old people is a personal responsibility to be carried out by kin. Sheila Neysmith and Lillian Wells argue that the evidence to support this claim is the plethora of policy statements which emphasize the role of public services as supporters or substitutes for family care.[40] From the very beginning, discussions around long-term-care reform have asserted that the family "is a key part of the delivery system."[41] As early as 1977, members of the then Conservative government were reportedly arguing that they would like to see families take responsibility for their elderly.[42] The Liberal white paper, *A New Agenda*, clearly states that "while government must provide leadership and facilitate necessary changes, the development of appropriate responses has to involve the co-operation and assistance of all elements of our society.[43] What we really want is a commitment from the municipalities and from the families that all of us are working carefully together."[44] Mavis Wilson made the Liberal stance on the issue perfectly clear when she stated that "families have the prime responsibility for caring" for their members. "It is the role of the government to assist families to be able to do their job. It is not my contention that the government should in any way replace the family. What we can do is empower families to care for their members."[45] Similarly, during the debates surrounding Bill 74, The Advocacy Act, in 1989, Steven Mahoney voiced his concern that the government not initiate a policy which could possibly "displace the family from what clearly is its rightful position ... it must be responsible." He added, "The role of the family shall be paramount."[46] This is not surprising given that one of the main goals of the Liberal's program of long-term-care reform was to strengthen the role of the local community in order to support family caregivers.[47]

NDP parliamentarians, meanwhile, insisted that "the government is neither expecting nor forcing family members and friends to become caregivers."[48] Nevertheless, party members asserted that families "have an important role to play" in community care.[49] This role was seen to be so important to the long-term care system proposed by the NDP that the ONHA stated that the party's policy seemed to be based upon "the assumption that families can and will do more and that old values around the family and care of the elderly will re-emerge as important social filters in coming years."[50] The association also cautioned that, when family care substitutes for the care of a professional, a degree of risk is involved.[51] It is dangerous to assume that family members are capable of providing the types of care many aged people require.[52]

Many seniors and their families were also quick to voice concerns that, despite government statements to the contrary, community care may in fact be part of an large-scale abdication by the state of its responsibility for care of the aged, leaving families with no choice but to provide the services the government is no longer willing to provide. Various seniors organizations have noted that dollars taken from the institutional sector were not always reallocated to home-care services. Jane Leitch of the Ontario Seniors Alliance reported in 1993 that in the community-care realm there had been no reform, redirection, or redeployment of resources. Instead, all that happened was that components of the existing system were dismantled or reduced in scope without the enhancement or growth of the community-based sector.[53] Funds promised by the state never actually surfaced as actual expenditures.[54]

As of May 1993, of the $640 million pledged to long-term care, only $100 million had been provided and only $26 million had actually been spent on the expansion of home-care services.[55] As a result, many seniors found that the community-care services they had hoped would be available to them were in fact not there. It seemed that families would either be forced to provide the services that were not being offered within the community or aged people would go without.[56]

The families of the aged had only to look to the families of mentally disabled children to see that the rhetoric of de-institutionalization and community care meant in practice that families ended up bearing most of the burden of caregiving. Anne Bullock has argued that, despite claims that care in the community would be more humane and that it was the best form of care for mentally disabled children, the Ontario government merely used the ideology of community care to expedite its own fiscal and administrative priorities.[57] The unpaid labour of family members was a vital and necessary component of the government's plan to reduce costs by removing the mentally disabled from institutions. Consequently, families bore the brunt of the state's requirement to divest itself of expensive long-term-care responsibilities.[58]

The NDP government's Bill 173, An Act Respecting Long-Term Care, gave the province the ability to override or opt out of certain sections of the Canada Health Act and restrict the benefits available under the Health Insurance Act.[59] The Conservative health critic, Cameron Jackson, claimed that the act gave Multiple Service Agencies (MSAs), which were to administer long-term care at the community level, the power to "make substantial decisions about people's lives as it relates to care and support in a home setting." Specifically, these agencies would be able to dictate which services a family received or did not receive to the point of deciding that they "get no service at all."[60] Basically, the government reserved the right to limit services to certain people or groups of people should financial constraints necessitate reducing the cost of long-term care programs. As Geoff Quirt, the acting executive director of the long-term care division of the Ministry of Health stated: "There is a finite amount of money available to spend on long-term care services in the community and in facilities and we have not claimed that everybody's demands will be met 100% to their satisfaction."[61]

Critics of the act argued that this "finite amount of money" would not be sufficient to operate community-based long-term-care programs at an adequate level. Liberal MPP Barbara Sullivan, for instance, questioned the accuracy of government financial predictions regarding the cost of long-term-care services, claiming that no reliable feasibility study or costing of MSAs had ever been carried out.[62] Similarly, Cameron Jackson argued that the government may have underestimated the costs involved in implementing and maintaining the proposed long-term-care programs.[63] It appears that community-based long-term-care programs would have been faced with financial difficulties within a very short time, if not from the moment they commenced operation.

The NDP's long-term-care policies were never implemented. In 1995, only months after Bill 173 was passed, the government was swept from office and the Conservative Party under Mike Harris was elected to power. Harris immediately made it clear that, although his party was committed to community-care programs, his party had no intention of proceeding with the reforms to long-term care outlined in Bill 173. A new Conservative policy was to be announced in the fall of 1995. As of the fall of 1996 there was still no formal statement concerning long-term care. However, there is little reason to believe that the Conservative reforms will increase spending on either institutional care or community-based programs, given the party's extreme emphasis on fiscal restraint. By December 1995 over $132 million had already been cut from the budget of the Ministry of Health alone. In total, Harris's government cut over $5.5 billion from the provincial budget in its first six months in office.

This turn of events raises the question of what will happen to community-care services in the future. If fiscal restraint becomes the guiding principal in long-term-care reform, as it has in almost every aspect of Conservative government policy, will services be removed from the list of caregiving activities funded by the state or will certain groups of people be declared ineligible for any services? It is not inconceivable that families will bear the brunt of any future spending or service reductions, in the sense that aged people living with kin may become the first group to have their services restricted. Hence, although the details are not yet clear, Conservative long-term-care reforms will likely reduce public spending on long-term care and thereby force families to do more. Indeed, it is almost certain that Conservative policies will contain an even greater potential than did NDP long-term-care reforms to enact a transfer of responsibility for the dependent aged from the state to the family.

In this regard, a discussion of the impact of community-care policies in Great Britain could prove useful. Unlike Ontario, where community-care programs remain too undeveloped and too new to be accurately evaluated, such policies have been in place in Britain since at least 1976[64] – long enough for their impact to have been studied and assessed. The British example can also offer a warning as to what can happen when fiscal restraint becomes the guiding principal for policy reforms. As Margot Jefferys explains, community care can mean different things to different people. Generally, community care is presented as part of the genuine desire of most populations to ensure that the aged are treated with dignity and that resources are made available to meet the needs of the frail and handicapped.[65] There is plenty of evidence in Great Britain, however, that under the Conservative government of Prime Minister Thatcher the will to implement these vague desires was deficient. As Janet Finch points out, "the history of community care to date appears to be characterized by an enthusiasm in rhetoric and in policy documents which has not been matched by a willingness to commit resources to the provision of the kinds of services which might facilitate its development. The gap between the rhetoric and the resources has been filled by volunteer and family labour."[66] In this sense, Finch argues, although the government presented community care as part of spectrum of services provided by the state, in reality community care came to mean not only care in the community but also care by the community. Further, research has demonstrated that care by the community, whether in England or Ontario, means that the provision of primary care falls not on the community as a whole but on specific groups and individuals, usually female family members.[67]

The British example also provides evidence that community-care rhetoric has the potential to become a means of reducing social-welfare expenditures.[68] Local authorities in Britain were instructed that, if they wished to lower levels of community expenditure, they needed to persuade families and the voluntary sector to take on some of the tasks previously carried out by social services.[69] In other words, one aim of emphasizing community care in Britain was the reduction of public expenditures by substituting younger kin and unpaid neighbourly support for paid professional services. The lesson is clear: the more desperately a government needs to reduce its funding, the more frequently families members will be forced to provide caregiving to the aged with little or no public support.

The British government does not consider itself responsible for providing care for those aged people who live with their families. In the allocation of community-based services, aged people who live alone are given priority while people who live with relatives have little access to such publicly provided support.[70] The state's responsibility is assumed to be essentially discharged if a person lives with a relative. Finch adds that, given the condition of public finances, it is likely that such trends will not only continue but accelerate, as residential services for the aged fail to expand while the aged population keeps on growing.[71]

Whether or not long-term-care reform in Ontario will follow a similar path is yet to be seen. Ontario has hardly reached the stage where the abdication of state responsibility for the aged is as obvious or as widespread as it is in Great Britain. Nevertheless, Ontario's long-term-care reforms are based on many of the same assumptions that guided nineteenth-century institutional-care policies. The previous chapters have demonstrated that many of those assumptions were inaccurate and the overall impact of policies based upon these assumptions was widespread suffering for the aged and their families. If long-term-care reform continues in its current direction, it is possible that a similar fate awaits today's elderly and their families.

Conclusion

This study began with the assertion that the state plays a central role in determining how individuals and society view the dependent aged and the family's obligations towards them. It was also argued that exactly what role the state has chosen to play has been determined by three factors: the degree of concern about the size of the aged population; beliefs about the level of need and dependency among that population; and the extent to which the state is concerned with fiscal restraint. In periods when the state fears a massive increase in the size of the aged population and also assumes that this population will be highly needy and dependent upon government for support, it is likely the state will attempt to reduce its responsibilities for this group. If such fears coincide with a period of fiscal restraint, it is almost certain that the state will abdicate a large portion of its responsibilities in this area and elect to emphasize family obligations in order to justify transferring these responsibilities to the family or the community. In periods of financial crisis, the image of the aged and their families put forward by the state often has more to do with justifying policy decisions than with providing an accurate image of the true circumstances of the elderly. It is also apparent that, when policy decisions concerning the aged are based upon the fiscal priorities of the state rather than the actual needs of the aged and their families, everyone involved suffers.

During the 1890s legislators were concerned with increases in the number of aged people in the population. While it was true that the aged population was growing, in actual fact the over-sixty population was growing at a slower rate than it had been in previous decades. It appears that government officials exaggerated the degree to which population aging was creating a problem in order to justify policies of fiscal restraint aimed at the dependent elderly. Similarly, although it cannot be denied that current populations are indeed aging, recent government reports have tended to exaggerate both the pace and the degree at which the size of Ontario's elderly population is growing. This may be due to factors completely unrelated to the elderly. In Great Britain and the United States, it has been shown that concern over the number of old people in society often has no connection to any actual change in the size of the aged population.

In Ontario, anxiety over the size of the aged population had more to do with the government's need to cut costs than with any real fear about population aging itself. In other words, in both the 1890s and the 1990s, the growing size of the aged population would not have attracted much attention in the legislature had it not been for the fact that in these periods the government faced a fiscal crisis.[1] In response, governments reduced the portion of the provincial budget allocated for social spending. As Samuel Resnick explains, depressions and hard economic times have generally encouraged governments to adopt less charitable attitudes towards the poor and to re-evaluate the degree of responsibility they wish to assume for dependent members of certain groups such as the elderly.[2] As one of most visible groups in receipt of government support, the dependent aged became one of the main targets of policies aimed at reducing government expenditures. In Ontario, during the 1890s as well as the 1990s, it was a reduction in spending on institutional care in particular that had the greatest impact upon the dependent elderly and their families.

During the depression of the 1890s government officials decided that, instead of increasing the space available in institutions to keep up with the growth of the aged population and the increasing poverty and need of their families, access to institutional care would be restricted to those old people with no relatives to care for them or to those aged individuals who were actually dangerous. One result was that aged people who had families, or who were senile but supposedly "easy to care for at home," found it increasingly difficult to gain admission into an insane asylum or house of refuge. Another was that families found themselves shouldered with an increasing burden of care as people once considered legitimate subjects of public institutional care became the sole obligation of their relatives.

Similarly, legislators in the early 1990s decided that institutional care for the elderly was too expensive. At the same time, government did not increase the capacity of institutional-care facilities despite a growing need for such services. Legislators argued that money spent on institutional care was wasted because "many seniors are institutionalized needlessly."[3] Instead, policy makers emphasized community care. Echoing the sentiments of their nineteenth-century predecessors, they insisted that a large portion of the present institutionalized aged population could be adequately cared for within their communities.

Officially, government has admitted its responsibility for supporting the network of community services which will be providing the care for those aged people no longer considered eligible for admission into institutions. Therefore, transferring the provision of services to the dependent elderly from institutions to the community may not necessarily represent a redefinition of state responsibilities into family obligations in the same way that government policies in the nineteenth century did. Yet there is reason to believe that, while long-term-care reform may not involve a drastic abdication of state responsibilities towards the aged, community-based care programs do possess the capacity to initiate a decrease in the level of support the provincial government provides for the dependent elderly. Future policy reforms could eventually force families to assume responsibilities that were, in many instances, formerly carried out by the state.

If this in indeed the case, the present study has demonstrated that Ontarians have cause to be concerned. Late-nineteenth-century government policies that attempted to redefine state responsibilities as family obligations had an overwhelmingly negative impact upon Ontario's aged population and their families. In most cases, by refusing to offer assistance to families attempting to care for ill or senile aged relatives, government officials placed upon families burdens which they were entirely unable to carry. The result was emotional and financial stress for families and widespread destitution and homelessness for the elderly. These problems occurred because policies that placed heavy burdens of responsibility for the aged on families were based upon inaccurate assumptions about the condition of the aged population and the level of care their families could provide.

The first assumption was that old age and dependency upon public resources were synonymous. In the 1890s there was little doubt in institutional administrators' minds that the bulk of the aged population was ill, senile, destitute, and dependent on public charity or on the care provided by government-funded houses of industry, houses of refuge, or asylums for the insane. These officials assumed that the old people found in provincial institutions were representative – in their poverty, illness, and isolation – of the entire aged population of the province. This assumption played a large role in convincing government officials that the boundary between state responsibilities and family obligations had to be redefined.

In reality, the institutionalized portion of the elderly population was exceptional in its poverty, illness, and dependency. As our study of Brockville's aged population demonstrated, the majority of the aged population was financially and physically capable of living independently. Those aged people who lacked the financial, physical, or mental resources to provide for themselves were often cared for by their family or friends. Less than 3 per cent of the total elderly population entered public institutions. This small minority of the population generally lacked relatives to care for them or required care that their families were sometimes unwilling but usually unable to provide.

Nevertheless, though the majority of the nineteenth-century aged population did not require government support, the assumption that all aged people were poor, ill, and dependent fuelled panic over population aging and the burden such trends represented to public resources. The belief that each additional old person in the population would require care and support from the state convinced officials in the 1890s that it was necessary to reduce the level of state responsibility for the aged in order to prevent a fiscal catastrophe in the future. Arguing that it could not provide care for every old person in the province, the government reduced or eliminated public support for the minority of the aged population that was truly dependent.

Similar fears seem to be driving current policy decisions. Twentieth-century legislators, although they have had a more sophisticated and refined image of old age, remain convinced that "poverty provides the essential context for the lives of many elderly people."[4] The same legislators also believe that, as a result of their illness and dependency, the aged place "heavy demands on an already overburdened system."[5] As in the nineteenth century, it is the ill, old, and destitute portion of the aged population, those most frequently in need of public support and care, who are seen to represent the aged population as a whole. This is so despite the fact that ample evidence exists to demonstrate that the majority of the senior citizens in Canada are capable of providing for their own needs. Less than one-third of the aged population, even those over the age of eighty-five, require the prolonged, complex, and expensive types of care that cause governments to panic. Yet, like nineteenth-century legislators, current government officials have decided that because the state cannot provide support for the entire aged population, it must reduce the amount of care it provides to those who most need it.

The next assumption that guided nineteenth-century policy makers was that Ontario's families were not providing a sufficient amount of care for their aged relatives. It was argued that institutions were being filled with old people mainly because their families were shirking their responsibilities and that when it came to the care of the aged there was a growing tendency among Ontarian families to "foist them upon the Government." This belief permitted legislators to maintain that there was no reason for the state to assume responsibilities that were properly family obligations. Seen from this perspective, restricting access to institutional care for those aged people who had relatives to care for them was not an abdication of state responsibilities but merely a method of returning the burden of caring for the aged to the family, where it rightly belonged.

In fact, however, nineteenth-century families provided massive amounts of care for their aged kin. Rather than abandoning the aged in institutions at the first possible moment, spouses, children, siblings, and other relatives generally did all they could to care for ill or senile elderly people and institutionalized them only when all alternatives had been exhausted. As a study of the case files of the Rockwood asylum reveals institutionalization was a desperate last resort rather than a convenient way to get rid of burdensome individuals. In several cases, the aged people who arrived at Rockwood required care that was well beyond the capacity of their families.

In the 1990s, long-term-care policies that emphasize care within the community also focus upon the role of the family. Considering that recent studies have demonstrated that 90 per cent of the care provided for the elderly occurs within the family,[6] provincial officials have been careful not to blame families directly for the rising numbers of seniors placed in institutions. Nevertheless, by arguing that a large portion of the institutionalized population really should not be there, legislators are suggesting that family members could care for these people but have chosen not to. It is also clear that, as stated officially, community care will rely on the involvement and cooperation of family members in the provision of services. Yet government spending cuts may mean that community care programs will not have sufficient resources to provide adequate care for every old person who requires it.[7] If this occurs, it is almost certain that public resources will be focused upon the portion of the aged population that has no relatives. As in the nineteenth century, aged people with no one to care for them will still be considered legitimate candidates for government support, while those old people with relatives will be viewed as the responsibility of their families.

Policies of this type assume that those dependent old people deemed ineligible for public support will be adequately cared for by their families. Evidence from the nineteenth century demonstrates that this assumption is not accurate. The Rockwood case files indicate that, when ill and senile old people were ejected from the institution on the assumption that their families could "easily" care for them at home, both the aged and their families suffered. The aged in question did not receive the care they required and their families found themselves unable to cope with the demands of providing amounts and types of care that were more than an average family could be expected to supply. Many of the families who sent their aged relatives to the asylum simply did not have the emotional, physical, or financial resources necessary to continue caring for them. This situation was made all the more unbearable by the fact that, throughout the nineteenth century, various provincial governments had refused to provide funding for communal support networks, thus destroying the traditional forms of assistance that had helped families cope with the care of their dependent relatives.

More recently, groups such as the Ontario Nursing Home Association have voiced concern that families in the 1990s may be no better able to cope with the demands of providing care for the ill or senile. They have demonstrated that a large portion of the old people in institutions require amounts and types of care that are beyond the capacity of most families. It is also likely that, if future governments enact fiscal-restraint policies that further restrict the growth of institutional facilities, there will soon be room in institutions for only those aged people exhibiting the most extreme forms of illness or derangement. This will mean that community services and families will be expected to care for people suffering from increasingly severe forms of mental and physical debility. As government officials have already stated, funds for community-care programs are limited. Therefore, it seems improbable that funding to community programs will be increased to match the increasingly complicated levels of care these programs will be expected to provide. While families coping with aged members suffering from the most severe illnesses may remain eligible for support from community services, it is almost certain that support for families caring for aged kin with less severe illnesses will be reduced or eliminated as the limited public funds allocated for these services are exhausted. In a manner similar to that of the nineteenth century, a lack of funding for community services may leave many families caring for dependent aged people without the very types of support that were supposed to help them cope with their caregiving responsibilities. Since this situation created widespread hardship in the 1890s, there is reason to fear that it will do likewise in the 1990s.

Why have policy makers allowed their decisions on care for the aged to be guided by erroneous information? Have legislators been unaware of the contradictions between the statements made by government officials concerning the situation of the province's aged population and their families and the true state of these people, or have they simply been uninterested in the truth since "the facts" might interfere with the implementation of their policies of fiscal restraint?

During the 1890s the government made statements concerning the growth of the institutionalized aged population and the irresponsibility of their families despite the fact that legislators had access to information which proved that many of these claims were false. The government presented the rising numbers of institutionalized elderly as evidence of a widespread lack of concern for the aged on the part of their families. In turn, these figures were employed as justification for reductions in public spending on the aged. Officials argued that such actions were necessary to recreate a sense of proper filial affections among the relatives of older people. Yet the evidence found in the case files of the Rockwood asylum and statements printed in the asylum's official reports indicate that the government was aware that families were not abandoning the aged. It appears that government officials purposely presented information in a manner that made families appear more irresponsible than they were.

While it is easy to see why officials would initially feel that the rising portion of aged people found inside institutions was a clear sign that families were shirking their responsibilities, it is doubtful that these administrators did not realize the truth. The government of the period was obsessed with tabulating facts and figures concerning such issues as population growth and rates of institutionalization. Census figures were available to policy makers and various agencies were well aware of growth among different segments of the population. It is hard to imagine that government officials were not also aware that the increase in the number of old people in provincial institutions did not indicate that rates of institutionalization among the aged were actually rising. These officials did know, however, that statistics and figures could be used to support any argument one wishes to advance.[8] Government reports and institutional administrators, for instance, repeatedly emphasized that admission rates among the elderly were increasing without mentioning the concurrent growth in the size of the aged population as a whole. In addition, admission figures and age breakdowns among institutional populations were used to create the impression that families were using institutions to get rid of troublesome aged individuals at public expense.[9]

This rhetoric served the purpose of justifying the government's cost-cutting measures, particularly the abdication of its responsibility for the aged. In other words, the government, rather than painting a true picture of the circumstances of the aged and their families, chose to present information in a manner that supported its ultimate goal of transforming state responsibilities into family ones. Government policies, in short, were aimed at reducing government spending, not doing what was best for the elderly population of the province. Justifying reductions in spending upon institutional care by arguing that families were not providing a sufficient amount of care for the aged and that they should, therefore, provide more ignored the fact that families were already providing as much care as they could. The end result of forcing families to supply more care for the dependent aged than they were capable of providing was that many aged people were simply left without adequate care.

To a lesser, but still significant, degree, policy makers in the 1990s have initiated reforms in long-term care to help reduce government spending on programs for the dependent aged rather than to ensure that this population receives adequate levels of care. One of the government's main justifications for shifting the provision of services from institutional settings into the community is the argument that these reforms are what the province's senior citizens have asked for. This information, legislators claim, was revealed in the public consultations the government carried out prior to enacting long-term-care reform. People involved in the consultations, however, have argued that "many of the questions raised at those public hearings do not in any way, shape or form reflect the vision that is set out in legislation terms."[10] It seems the government may have chosen to act upon only that portion of the data gathered at the public hearings which reflected its predetermined objectives – objectives that may have had more to do with fiscal restraint than with the provision of needed services.[11]

In addition, the government has argued that community services will reduce expenditures while maintaining an adequate level of care. Information in various studies would suggest that this is not possible. The government, however, has chosen to avoid the entire issue by not investigating the validity of its assumptions. No government studies have been done to prove that community-care programs are less costly than institutional care, or that community services will be able to provide adequate levels of care to the ill and senile aged population. As well, various groups have expressed serious concerns that the funds dedicated to the provision of community-care services are inadequate. Overall, it appears that fiscal objectives rather than the real needs of the aged population have played the major role in dictating the nature of recent long-term-care reforms.

In both the 1890s and the early 1990s, the provincial government was concerned about the growing numbers of aged people in the population. The truth was, however, that the actual number of aged people in the province was not the true reason for this concern. What alarmed government officials in both periods was the burden on the state treasury that these aged people were seen to represent. This fear was based on the equation of old age with dependency. It was assumed that elderly people necessarily represented a tax upon the resources of the government. In and of itself, however, even this assumption was not enough to spark panic. Rather, panic was created by the fact that population aging was occurring at the same time as a major economic crisis. The 1890s, like the 1990s, was a period of depression and declining government revenues. Fiscal restraint was as much a priority for late-nineteenth-century governments as it was for late-twentieth-century ones. When forced to cut costs, both governments looked to the dependent aged and re-evaluated the degree of responsibility the state wished to assume for this group. This involved reducing the number of aged people housed in or eligible for care in provincially funded institutions.

In the 1890s the state reduced spending on institutional care for the aged by emphasizing family obligations and forcing family members to care for their ill and senile elderly relatives. In the 1990s the government emphasized community care rather than family obligations as a means of reducing the number of aged people housed in provincial institutions. Yet it is clear that the community care described in the NDP government's long-term-care legislation involved a major increase in the degree of care to be provided by family members.

The policies of the Ontario's late-nineteenth-century government would not, in theory, have created undue hardships for either the dependent elderly or their families if they had in fact been a true response to actual conditions. Unfortunately, these policies were not based upon what was best for the aged; instead, they were enacted to help the government achieve its goals of fiscal restraint. The fact that current government legislation has much in common with that of the nineteenth century should create concern that it, too, rests on inaccurate assumptions about the aged population, the burden they represent to public resources, and the role their families should play in their care. If this is the case, the public should also recognize that modern-day policies may have the same negative impact upon the elderly as nineteenth-century ones did.

Current reforms to long-term care have the potential to provide a wide range of much needed services to a large segment of Ontario's aged population and their families. Unfortunately, these policy reforms also establish the framework for what could become a major redefinition of the role the state is willing to play in the provision of services to the elderly portion of the population. Exactly how these programs are implemented and maintained in the future will determine what the ultimate impact of long-term-care reform will be. Lessons from the past indicate that, if fiscal restraint becomes the primary motivation behind the implementation of reforms, it is highly probable that families will be forced to shoulder an increasing share of the burden of providing care for their ill, disabled, or senile elderly relatives. In this sense, if the funds provided for community-care programs are inadequate or are reduced to meet financial objectives, long-term-care reform will become the means by which state responsibilities are transformed into family obligations. The experience of the 1890s should warn legislators that such a redistribution of responsibility will almost certainly have a negative effect on a large segment of Ontario's population.

Notes

ABBREVIATIONS

AO   Archives of Ontario

AR   *Annual Report of the Inspector of Prisons and Public Charities for the Province of Ontario* (year appears in brackets)
Where the reference is to a particular report, particularly on asylums, the specific institution appears in brackets: for example, AR (1898): (Rockwood).

CTA   City of Toronto Archives

MU   Manuscript Collection

NAC   National Archives of Canada

RG   Record Group

INTRODUCTION

1 David Thomson, *Selfish Generations? How Welfare States Grow Old* (Wellington, New Zealand: White Horse Press 1996), 215–16.

2 Ibid., 215–40, provides an excellent discussion of this point.

3 See Pat Thane, "The Growing Burden of an Aging Population?" *Journal of Public Policy,* vol. 7, no. 4 (Oct.–Dec. 1987): 373–87, 376; James Franke, "Support for Aging Policy: Self-Interest, Social Justice and Political Symbols," *Journal of Aging Studies,* vol. 1, no. 4 (winter 1987): 393–406, 393.

4 Robert Evans, "Reading the Menu With Better Glasses: Aging and Health Policy Research," in *Aging and Health: Linking Research and Public Policy,* ed. S.J. Lewis (Chelsea, Michigan: 1987): 145–67, 146; see also Margot Jefferys, "The Over-Eighties in Britain: The Social Construction of Panic," *Journal of Public Health Policy,* vol. 4 (1983): 367–72, 368.

5 Clyde Hertzman and Michael Hayes, "Will the Elderly Really Bankrupt Us with Increased Health Care Costs," *Canadian Journal of Public Health*, vol. 76 (1985): 373–7, 373–5.

6 Elizabeth Binney and Carroll Estes, "The Retreat of the State and Its Transfer of Responsibility: The Intergenerational War," *International Journal of Health Services*, vol. 18, no. 1 (1988): 83–96, 83; Carroll Estes, "The Reagan Legacy: Privatization, The Welfare State and Aging in the 1990's," in *The State, Labour Markets and the Future of Old Age Policy*, ed. John Myles and Jill Quadagno (Philadelphia, PA: Temple University Press 1991): 59–83, 76; Janet Finch, *Family Obligations and Social Change* (Cambridge, U.K.: Polity Press 1989), 2–7.

7 See A. Pollett, I. Anderson, and P. O'Connor, "For Better or Worse: The Experience of Caring for an Elderly Dementing Spouse," *Ageing and Society*, vol. 11 (1991): 443–69, 443–4; Carroll Estes, Robert Newcomer *et al.*, *Fiscal Austerity and Aging: Shifting Government Responsibility for the Elderly* (London: Sage Publications 1983), 20; Meredith Minkler, "Blaming the Aged Victim: The Politics of Scapegoating in Times of Fixed Conservation," *International Journal of Health Services*, vol. 13 (1983): 155–68, 155; William Graebner, "A Comment: The Social Security Crisis in Perspective," in *Old Age in a Bureaucratic Society: The Elderly, The Experts and American Historians*, ed. David Van Tassel and Peter Stearns (Westport, Conn.: Greenwood Press 1986): 217–21, 219.

8 Estes, Newcomer *et al.*, *Fiscal Austerity and Aging*, 21; Jill Quadagno, "Generational Equity and the Politics of the Welfare State," *International Journal of Health Services*, vol. 20, no. 4 (1990): 631–50, 631.

9 Carroll Estes, "The Reagan Legacy," 63; Estes, Newcomer *et al*, *Fiscal Austerity and Aging*, 21.

10 Carroll Estes, "The Reagan Legacy," 71–6; Binney and Estes, "The Retreat of the State," 83.

11 Janet Finch, *Family Obligations*, 2–7, and Margot Jefferys, "The Over-Eighties in Britain: The Social Construction of Panic," *Journal of Public Health Policy*, vol. 4 (1983): 367–72, 368. Also, see Allan Walker, "Thatcherism and the New Politics of Old Age," in Myles and Quadagno (eds.), *States, Labor Markets and Old Age Policy*, 19–35.

12 Leroy Stone and Michael MacLean, *Future Income Prospects for Canada's Senior Citizens* (Toronto: Institute for Research on Public Policy 1979), iii, 33.

13 Thomas Walkom, "Pensions will be battleground in attack on elderly," *Toronto Star*, 8 Sept. 1994, A-25.

14 Susan Watt, "Models of Family in Health Policy for the Aged," *Canadian Review of Social Policy*, vol. 25 (May 1990): 33–46, 33.

15 See Sheila Neysmith and Lillian Wells, "Home Care: Who Defines the Priorities," in *An Aging Population: The Challenge for Community Action*, ed. Lillian Wells (Toronto: University of Toronto Press 1991): 96–107, 102.

16 Thomson, *Selfish Generations?* 67.

17 Ibid., 72.

18 Ibid., 22–4.

19 For two of the more recent examples, see Alan Walker, "The Future of Long-Term Care in Canada: A British Perspective," *Canadian Journal on Aging*, vol. 14, no. 2 (summer 1995): 437–46, and Raisa Deber and Paul Williams, "Policy, Payment and Participation: Long-Term Care Reform in Ontario," *Canadian Journal on Aging*, vol. 14, no. 2 (summer 1995): 294–318. Also, see Rosalie Kane and Robert Kane, "Home and Community Based Care in Canada," in *Financing Home Care: Improving Protection for the Disabled Elderly*, ed. Diane Rowland and Barbara Lyons (Baltimore, Md.: 1991).

20 Thomson, *Selfish Generations?* 29.

21 Finch, *Family Obligations and Social Change*, 57.

22 Jane Aronson, "Family Care of the Elderly: Underlying Assumptions and Their Consequences," *Canadian Journal on Aging*, vol. 4, no. 3 (1985): 115–25, 121.

23 David Thomson, "Welfare and Historians," in *The World We Have Gained*, ed. L. Bonfield, R. Smith, and K. Wrightson (New York: Basil Blackwell 1986): 355–78, 357; Carole Haber and Brian Gratton, "Aging in America: The Perspective of History," in *Handbook of the Humanities and Aging*, ed. Thomas Cole, David Van Tassel, and Robert Kastenbaum (New York: Springer Press 1992): 352–70, 353; Linda Gordon, "Social Insurance and Public Assistance: The Influence of Gender in Welfare Thought in the United States, 1890–1935," *American Historical Review*, vol. 97, no. 1 (February 1992): 19–54, 37.

24 Jill Quadagno, "The Transformation of Old Age Security," in Van Tassel and Stearns (eds.), *Old Age in a Bureaucratic Society*, 129–52, 150.

25 See Allan Walker, "The Social Creation of Poverty and Dependency in Old Age," *Journal of Social Policy*, vol. 9 (1980): 45–75, 49; Allan Walker, "Pensions and the Production of Poverty in Old Age, 1970's–1980's," in *Ageing and Social Policy: A Critical Assessment*, ed. C. Phillips and Allan Walker (London: Aldershot 1986); Peter Townsend, "The Structured Dependency of the Elderly: A Creation of Social Policy in the Twentieth Century," *Ageing and Society*, vol. 1 (1981): 5–28, 23; Peter Townsend, "Ageism and Social Policy," in Walker and Philips, (eds.), *Ageing and Social Policy*, 15–41. Also, see Brian Gratton, "Labour Force Participation of Older Men, 1890–1950," *Journal of Social History*, vol. 20 (1987): 689–710, for a review of similar trends in American policy.

26 Townsend, "The Structured Dependency of the Elderly," 23.

27 John Myles, "The Aged, The State and the Structure of Inequality," in *Structured Inequality in Canada*, ed. John Harp and John Hofley (Scarborough, Ont.: Prentice Hall 1980): 317–42, 323.

28 Finch, *Family Obligations,* 139.

29 Ibid., 115.

30 Ibid., 10.

31 Ibid., 243.

32 Thomson, *Selfish Generations?* 114–15.

33 Watts, "Models of Family in Health Policy for the Aged," 38.

34 See Brian Gratton, *Urban Elders: Family, Work and Welfare Among Boston's Aged, 1890–1950* (Philadelphia, PA: Temple University Press 1986), and Jill Quadagno, *Aging in Early Industrial Society: Work, Family and Social Policy in Nineteenth-Century England* (New York: Academic Press 1982).

35 Herbert Northcott, *Aging in Alberta: Rhetoric and Reality* (Calgary: Detselig 1992), 87; Sheila McIntyre, "Old Age As a Social Problem: Historical Notes on the English Experience," in *Health Care and Health Knowledge,* ed. D. Dingwall, C. Heath, and M. Ried (London, Croom Helm 1977): 41–63, 42. Also, see Janet Roebuck and Jane Slaughter, "Ladies and Pensioners: Stereotypes and Public Policy Affecting Old Women in England, 1880–1940," *Journal of Social History,* vol. 13, no. 1 (fall 1979): 105–114.

36 McIntyre, "Old Age as a Social Problem," 42. Also, see Estes, Newcomer *et al., Fiscal Austerity and Aging,* 14.

37 Northcott, *Aging in Alberta,* 88.

38 Susan McDaniel, "Demographic Aging As a Guiding Paradigm in Canada's Welfare State," *Canadian Public Policy,* vol. 13, no. 3 (1987): 330–6, 331.

39 Northcott, *Aging in Alberta,* 5.

40 Ibid., 4.

41 Ellen Gee, "Historical Change in the Family Life-Course of Canadian Men and Women," in *Aging in Canada,* ed. Victor Marshall (Markham, Ont.: Fitzhenry and Whiteside 1987): 265–87, 265.

42 Judith Husbeck, *Old and Obsolete: Age Discrimination and the American Worker, 1860–1920* (New York: Garamond 1989), 10.

43 "We're growing older faster and StatsCan is concerned," *Ottawa Citizen,* 24 Jan. 1995, A–25.

44 Sara Arber and Jay Ginn, "The Invisibility of Age: Gender and Class in Later Life," *Sociological Review,* vol. 39, no. 2 (May 1991): 260–91, 263–4.

45 Northcott, *Aging in Alberta,* 4.

46 Thomas Walkom, "Pensions will be battleground."

47 Christopher Conrad, "Old Age in the Modern and Postmodern Western World," in Cole, Van Tassel, and Kaskerbaum (eds.), *Handbook of the Humanities and Aging,* 82; and Shegog, *Impending Crisis of Old Age,* 4.

48 Northcott, *Aging in Alberta,* 1.

49 See W.R. Bytheway, "Demographic Statistics and Old Age Ideology," *Ageing and Society,* vol. 3, no. 3 (November 1981): 347–64; and Estes, Newcomer *et al., Fiscal Austerity and Aging,* 18.

50 See Stephen Katz, "Alarmist Demography: Power, Knowledge and the Elderly Population," *Journal of Aging Studies*, vol. 6, no. 3 (fall 1992): 203–25, 220; and Walker and Phillips (eds.), *Ageing and Social Policy*, introduction, II.

51 McDaniel, "Demographic Aging as a Guiding Paradigm," 331.

52 Fred Pampel and J.B. Williamson, "Welfare Spending in Advanced Industrial Democracies, 1950–1980," *American Journal of Sociology*, vol. 93, no. 6 (May 1988): 1,424–56, 1,449.

53 Finch, *Family Obligations*, 115.

54 Walker, "The Future of Long-Term Care in Canada," 444.

55 Neena Chappell, *About Canada: The Aging of the Canadian Population* (Ottawa: Department of the Secretary of State of Canada 1990), 31.

56 See Pat Thane, "The Debate on the Declining Birth-Rate in Britain: The 'Menace' of an Aging Population, 1920's-1950's," *Continuity and Change*, vol. 5 (1990): 283–305; and Peter Laslett, "Family, Kinship and Collectivity As Systems of Support in Pre-industrial Europe: A Consideration of the Nuclear Hardship Hypothesis," *Continuity and Change*, vol. 3, no. 2 (1988): 153–75.

57 Rod Mickleburg, "Silver threads threaten to strangle the system," *Globe and Mail*, 1 May 1992.

58 Hazel Qureshi and Allan Walker, "Caring for Elderly People: The Family and the State," in Phillips and Walker, (eds.), *Ageing and Social Policy*, 109–27, 110.

59 Bernice Neugarten and Dail Neugarten, "Changing Meanings of Age in the Aging Society," in *Our Aging Society: Paradox and Promise*, ed. Alan Pifer and Lydia Bonte (New York: Norton 1986): 33–51, 35–6; Finch, *Family Obligations*, 168.

60 Thane, "The Growing Burden of an Aging Population," 378.

61 M.S. Marzouk, "Aging, Age Specific Health Care Costs and the Future Health Care Burden in Canada," *Canadian Public Policy*, vol. 17, no. 4 (1991): 490–506, 502–3. Also, see Stephen Katz, "Alarmist Demographics: Power, Knowledge and the Elderly Population," *Journal of Aging Studies*, vol. 6, no. 3 (fall 1992): 203–25, 207; Evans, "Reading the Menu With Better Glasses"; and Hertzman and Hayes, "Will the Elderly Really Bankrupt Us," 375.

62 James Struthers, "The Provincial Welfare State: Social Policy in Ontario," *Journal of Canadian Studies*, vol. 27, no. 1 (spring 1992): 136–46, 137.

63 Ted Ball, "Lobbying Government for Long-Term Care," in *Long-Term Care in an Aging Society: Choices and Challenges for the 90's*, ed. Gerald Larue and Rich Bayly (New York: Golden Age Book 1992): 131–40.

64 *Globe*, "The Legislature," 25 March 1890, 1.

65 Aronson, "Family Care of the Elderly," 116.

66 Ann Shola Orloff, *The Politics of Pensions: A Comparative Analysis of Britain, Canada and the United States, 1880–1940* (Madison, WIS.: University

of Wisconsin Press 1993), 33; Also, see Richard Deaton, *The Political Economy of Pensions: Power, Politics and Social Change in Canada, Britain and the United States* (Vancouver: University of British Columbia Press 1989).

67 Tamera Hareven, "An Ambiguous Alliance: Some Aspects of American Influence on Canadian Social Welfare," *Histoire Sociale / Social History,* vol. 3 (1969): 82–98, 98.

68 Gordon Stewart, *The Origins of Canadian Politics: A Comparative Approach* (Vancouver: University of British Columbia Press 1986), 8 (see introduction and chapter 2).

69 Hareven, "An Ambiguous Alliance," 95.

70 See Judith Roebuck, "When does Old Age Begin: The Evolution of the English Definition," *Journal of Social History,* vol. 12 (1979): 416–28.

71 John Demos, "Old Age in Early New England," in *Aging, Death and the Completion of Being,* ed. David Van Tassel (Philadelphia, PA.: University of Pennsylvania Press 1986), 116.

72 David Radcliffe, "Growing Old in Ontario: A Grey Area," in *New Directions for the Study of Ontario's Past,* ed. David Gagan and Rosemary Gagan (Hamilton, Ont.: McMaster University Press 1988): 179–86, 86.

73 George Emery, "Ontario's Civil Registration of Vital Statistics, 1869–1926: The Evolution of an Administrative System," *Canadian Historical Review,* vol. 64, no. 4 (1983): 494–518, 494.

74 See Howard Chudacoff, *How Old Are You? Age Consciousness in American Culture* (Princeton, N.J.: Princeton University Press 1989).

75 See illustration in Jill Quadagno, *Aging in Early Industrial Society,* 111.

76 Michael Anderson, "The Impact on the Family Relationships of the Elderly of Changes, since Victorian Times, in Governmental Income Maintenance," in *Family, Bureaucracy and the Elderly,* ed. Ethel Shanas and Marvin Sussman (Durham, N.C.: Duke University Press 1977), 36–59, 40.

77 Roebuck, "When Does Old Age Begin," 418.

78 See Allan Walker, "Community Care and the Elderly in Great Britain: Theory and Practice," *International Journal of Health Services,* vol. 11, no. 4 (1981): 541–57, 541.

CHAPTER 1

1 Margaret Pelling and Richard Smith, "Introduction," in *Life, Death and the Elderly: Historical Perspectives,* ed. Margaret Pelling and Richard Smith (London: Routledge 1991), 7.

2 Stephen Smith, "Death, Dying and the Elderly in Seventeenth-Century England," in *Aging and the Elderly: Humanistic Perspectives in Gerontology,* ed. S. Spiker, K. Woodwood, and D. Van Tassel (Atlantic Highlands, N.J.: Humanities Press 1978), 205.

3 Peter Laslett, "Family, Kinship and the Collectivity As Systems of Support in Pre-industrial Europe: A Consideration of the Nuclear-Hardship Hypothesis," *Continuity and Change*, vol. 3, no. 2 (1988): 153–75, 168. Also, see Pat Thane, "The Debate on the Declining Birth Rate in Britain: The 'Menace' of an Aging Population," *Continuity and Change*, vol. 5 (1990): 283–305, 283.

4 Peter Stearns, *Old Age in European Society: The Case of France* (New York: Holmes Meier 1976), 19. See also David Thomson, "The Welfare of the Elderly in the Past: A Family or a Community Responsibility," in Pelling and Smith (eds.), *Life, Death and the Elderly*, 196.

5 David Troyansky, *Old Age in the Old Regime: Image and Experience in Eighteenth-Century France* (London: Cornell University Press 1989), 10.

6 John Demos, "Old Age in Early New England," in *Aging, Death and the Completion of Being*, ed. David Van Tassel (Philadelphia, PA.: University of Pennsylvania Press 1979), 131.

7 Demos, "Old Age in Early New England," 123.

8 Alfred Kutzik, "American Social Provision for the Aged: An Historical Perspective," in *Ethnicity and Aging*, ed. Donald Gelfand and Alfred Kutzik (New York: Springer 1979), 34.

9 J.B. Williamson, "Old Age Relief Policies Prior to 1900: The Trend Towards Restrictiveness," *American Journal of Economics and Sociology*, vol. 43, no. 3 (1984): 369–84, 371.

10 Demos, "Old Age in Early New England," 123.

11 David Hackett Fischer, *Growing Old in America* (New York: Oxford University Press 1977), 245.

12 Ibid., 3.

13 Carole Haber, *Beyond Sixty-Five: The Dilemma of Old Age in America's Past* (Cambridge, U.K.: Cambridge University Press 1983), 8.

14 Roger Ramson and Richard Sutch, "The Labour of Older Americans: Retirement of Men on and off the Job, 1870–1937," *Journal of Economic History*, vol. 46 (1986): 1–30, 16; Peter Laslett, "The Traditional English Family and the Aged in Our Society," in Van Tassel (ed.), *Aging, Death and the Completion of Being*, 99; and Smith, "Death, Dying and the Elderly."

15 Jacques Vallin, "Mortality in Europe from 1720 to 1914: Long-Term Trends and Changes in Patterns by Age and Sex," in *The Decline of Mortality in Europe*, ed. R. Schofield, R. Reher, and A. Bideau (Oxford, U.K.: Claraden Press 1991): 38–67, 49–54; Demos, "Old Age in Early New England," 131; and Troyansky, *Old Age in the Old Regime*, 10.

16 George Emery and Kevin McQuillan, "A Case Study Approach to Ontario Mortality History: The Example of Ingersol, 1881–1972," *Canadian Studies in Population*, vol. 15, no. 2 (1988): 135–58, 151.

17 Peter Laslett, "The History of Aging and the Aged," in *Family Life and Illicit Love in Earlier Generations: Essays in Historical Sociology* (Cambridge, U.K.: Cambridge University Press 1977), 189.

18 Howard Chudacoff, *How Old Are You?: Age Consciousness in American Culture* (Princeton, N.J.: Princeton University Press 1989), 11.

19 Laurel Thatcher Ulrich, *Good Wives: Image and Reality in the Lives of Women in New England, 1650–1750* (New York: Alfred Knopf 1982), 148–9.

20 See Demos, "Old Age in Early New England."

21 Sheila McIntyre, "Old Age As a Social Problem: Historical Notes on the English Experience," in *Health Care and Health Knowledge*, ed. R. Dingwall, C. Heath, and M. Reid (London: Croom Helm 1977): 41–63, 43. Also, see Peter Wood, *Poverty and the Workhouse in Victorian Britain* (Wolteboro Falls, N.H.: Allan Sutton 1991), 31, 113.

22 Jill Quadagno, *Aging in Early Industrial Society: Work, Family and Policy in Nineteenth-Century England* (New York: Academic Press 1982), 200.

23 Thane, "The Debate on the Declining Birth Rate in Britain," 283–305.

24 Ibid., 305.

25 See Stephen Katz, "Alarmist Demography: Power, Knowledge and the Elderly Population," *Journal of Aging Studies*, vol. 6, no. 3 (fall 1992): 203–25.

26 W.R. Bytheway, "Demographic Statistics and Old Age Ideology," *Ageing and Society*, vol. 1, no. 3 (November 1981): 347–64, 347.

27 John Myles, *Old Age in the Welfare State: The Political Economy of Public Pensions* (Toronto: Brown 1984), 104.

28 Katz, "Alarmist Demography," 206.

29 See Carole Haber and Brian Gratton, *Old Age and the Search for Security: An American Social History* (Bloomington, Ind.: University of Indiana Press 1994), 65.

30 Quadagno, *Aging in Early Industrial Society*, 87, and Michael Anderson, "The Impact on the Family Relationships of the Elderly of Changes, since Victorian Times, in Governmental Income Maintenance," in *Family, Bureaucracy and the Elderly*, ed. Ethel Shanas and Marvin Sussman (Durham, N.C.: 1977): 36–59.

31 Demos, "Old Age in Early New England," 141.

32 S.J. Wright, "The Elderly and the Bereaved in Eighteenth-Century Ludlow," in Pelling and Smith (eds.), *Life, Death and the Elderly*, 102–34, 102.

33 Kutzik, "American Social Provision for the Aged," 34.

34 David Thomson, "Welfare and Historians," in *The World We Have Gained*, ed. L. Bonfield, R. Smith, and K. Wrightson (New York: Basil Blackwell 1986), 355–78, 361; and David Thomson, "The Welfare of the Elderly in the Past: A Family of Community Responsibility," in Pelling and Smith (eds.), *Life, Death and the Elderly*, 194–22, 206.

35 Richard Smith, "The Manorial Court and the Elderly Tenant in Late Medieval England," in ibid., 39–61, 22.

36 See, for example, Thomson, "Welfare and Historians"; David Thomson, "I Am Not My Father's Keeper": Families and the Elderly in Nineteenth-

Century England," *Law and History Review*, vol. 2, no. 2 (fall 1984), 265–86; Thomson, "The Welfare of the Elderly in the Past"; and Richard Smith, "The Structured Dependency of the Elderly As a Recent Development: Some Sceptical Historical Thoughts," *Ageing and Society*, vol. 4, no. 4 (1984): 409–28.

37 See Gary Nash, "Poverty and Poor Relief in Pre-revolutionary Philadelphia," *William and Mary Quarterly*, vol. 33 (January 1976): 3–30; Raymond Mohl, "Poverty in Early America, A Reappraisal: The Case of Eighteenth-Century New York City," *New York History*, vol. 50 (1969): 5–27; and Seamus Metress, "The History of Irish-American Care of the Aged," *Social Services Review*, vol. 59, no. 1 (March 1985): 18–51.

38 Judith Husbeck, *Old and Obsolete: Age Discrimination and the American Worker, 1860–1920* (New York: Garland Press 1989), 1.

39 See W. Andrew Achenbaum, *Old Age in a New Land* (Baltimore, Md.: Johns Hopkins University Press 1978), 66–75; W. Andrew Achenbaum, "The Obsolescence of Old Age in America in America, 1865–1914," *Journal of Social History*, vol. 8 (fall 1974): 48–62, 56; William Graebner, *A History of Retirement: The Meaning and Function of an American Institution, 1885–1978* (New Haven, Conn.: Yale University Press 1980), 10–14; Carole Haber, "Mandatory Retirement in Nineteenth-Century America: The Conceptual Basis for a New Work Cycle," *Journal of Social History*, vol. 12 (fall 1978); 77–96.

40 Graebner, *A History of Retirement*, 58.

41 Achenbaum, "Obsolescence of Old Age," 56. Also, see Graebner, *A History of Retirement*, 12 (he cites Achenbaum).

42 Margaret Pelling, "Old Age, Poverty and Disability in Early Modern Norwich: Work, Remarriage and Other Expedients," in Pelling and Smith (eds.), *Life, Death and the Elderly*, 74–101, 79.

43 Brian Gratton, "The New Welfare State: Security and Retirement in 1950," *Social Science History*, vol. 12, no. 2 (summer 1988): 171–96, 172; Brian Gratton, *Urban Elders: Family, Work and Welfare Among Boston's Aged, 1890–1950* (Philadelphia, PA.: Temple University Press 1986), 61.

44 Howard Chudacoff and Tamera Hareven, "From the Empty Nest to Family Dissolution: Life-Course Transitions into Old Age," *Journal of Family History*, vol. 4, no. 1 (spring 1977), 69–82, 74.

45 Sara Arber and Jay Ginn, "The Invisibility of Age: Gender and Class in Later Life," *Sociological Review*, vol. 39, no. 2 (May 1991): 260–91, 270.

46 Sue Weiller, "Industrial Scrap-heap: Employment Patterns and Change for the Aged in the 1920's," *Social Science History*, vol. 13, no. 1 (spring 1989), 65–88, 66.

47 Sue Weiller, "Family Security of Social Security: The Family and the Elderly in New York State in the 1920's," *Journal of Family History*, vol. 11 (spring 1986): 77–95, 84.

48 Chudacoff and Hareven, "From Empty Nest to Family Dissolution," 228.

49 Haber, *Beyond Sixty-Five*, 34.

50 Gratton, *Urban Elders*, 175.

51 Roger Ramson and Richard Sutch, "The Decline of Retirement in the Years Before Social Security: United States Retirement Patterns, 1870–1940," in *Issues in Contemporary Retirement*, ed. R.R. Campbell and E. Lazear (Stanford, A.: Hoover Institution Press 1988): 3–37, 3.

52 Ramson and Sutch, "The Decline of Retirement," 6.

53 Ramson and Sutch, "The Labour of Older Americans," 5–6.

54 Ramson and Sutch, "The Decline of Retirement," 6.

55 Haber and Gratton, *Old Age and the Search for Security*, 105.

56 Ramson and Sutch, "The Decline of Retirement," 2.

57 See Ramson and Sutch, "The Labour of Older Americans."

58 Brian Gratton and Francis Rotondo, "Industrialization, the Family Economy and the Economic Status of the American Elderly," *Social Science History*, vol. 15 (1991): 337–62, 355. David Thomson suggests that savings were also a significant form of income for the elderly in England at this time; see Thomson, "The Welfare of the Elderly in the Past," 206.

59 See Ramson and Sutch, "The Decline of Retirement," 3, and Gratton and Rotondo, "Industrialization," 338. For further examples of aged people surviving by pooling the resources of the entire family, see Elycie Rotella and George Alter, "Working Class Debt in the Late-Nineteenth-Century United States," *Journal of Family History*, vol. 18, no. 2 (spring 1993): 111–34; Cheryl Elman, "Turn-of-the-Century Dependency and Interdependence: Roles of Teens in Family Economies of the Aged," *Journal of Family History*, vol. 18, no. 1 (winter 1993), 65–85; and Haber and Gratton, *Old Age and the Search for Security*, 69.

60 See Bentley Gilbert, "The Decay of Nineteenth-Century Provident Institutions and the Coming of Old Age Pensions in Great Britain," *Economic History Review*, vol. 17 (1964): 551–63.

61 Gratton and Rotondo, "Industrialization," 345.

62 Haber and Gratton, *Old Age and the Search for Security*, 66–79.

63 Andrew Scull, *Museums of Madness: The Social Organization of Insanity in Mid-Nineteenth-Century England* (London: A. Lane 1978), 40.

64 CTA, SC 35, series F: *Annual Report of the Toronto House of Industry* (Toronto 1866), 8.

65 CTA, SC 35, series H: "Continuation of Mayor's Annual Inspection," *Globe* 6 Feb. 1882.

66 CTA, SC 35, series H: "Our Christian Charities," Toronto *Empire Toronto*, 6 Nov. 1892.

67 CTA, SC 35, series H: "House of Industry," Toronto *Mail*, c. 1888.

68 CTA, SC 35, series F: *Annual Reports of the Toronto House of Industry* (see various reports between 1866 and 1899).

69 CTA, SC 35, series H: "Continuation of Mayor's Annual Inspection," *Globe*, 6 Feb. 1882.

70 Thomas Brown, "Living with God's Afflicted: A History of the Provincial Lunatic Asylum at Toronto, 1838–1911," Phd Thesis, Queen's University, 1980, 24; also, see AR (1893), appendix, 6.

71 AR (1897), "Report upon Common Gaols, Prisons and Reformatories". Also, see Richard Splane, *Social Welfare in Ontario, 1793–1893: A Study of Public Welfare Administration* (Toronto: University of Toronto Press 1965), 102.

72 Ibid., 102.

73 AR (1892), cited in the Prisoners' Aid Association of Canada, *County Paupers and County Houses of Industry* (Toronto: Dudley Press 1894), 16.

74 CTA: SC 35, series H: "Discussed Care of Aged Poor," *Mail and Empire*, 3 May 1898.

75 Brown, "Living with God's Afflicted," 108.

76 AO, RG 63, Records of the Inspector of Prisons and Public Charities, series A–1, envelope 24 (file 970), Dr Metcalfe to J.W. Langmuir (June 1879).

77 See case files of the Rockwood Asylum for the Insane in AO: RG 10, series F–20–1, especially cases 3,110 and 1,679.

78 Prisoners' Aid Association, *County Paupers*, 1.

79 Haber, *Beyond Sixty-Five*, 28–35, and Carole Haber, "And the Fear of the Poorhouse: Perceptions of Old Age Impoverishment in Early Twentieth-Century America," *Generations*, vol. 17, no. 2 (spring-summer 1993): 46–50, 46.

80 Testimony given to the House of Commons special committee on old age pensions between 1911 and 1913, cited in Kenneth Bryden, *Old Age Pensions and Policy Making in Canada* (Montreal: McGill-Queen's University Press 1974), 42.

81 Gratton, *Urban Elders*, 126. Also, see Richard Deaton, *The Political Economy of Pensions: Power, Politics and Social Change in Canada, Britain and the United States* (Vancouver: University of British Columbia Press 1989), 18; Haber and Gratton, *Old Age and Search for Security*, 127. For a more detailed analysis of the motives behind social workers' characterization of the aged as helpless and dependent, see Brian Gratton, "Social Workers and Old Age Pensions," *Social Services Review*, vol. 57 (1983): 403–15, 411.

82 Carole Haber, "From Senescence to Senility: The Transformation of Senile Old Age in the Nineteenth-Century," *Interdisciplinary Journal of Aging and Human Development*, vol. 19, no. 1 (1984–85), 41–5, 43–4; Haber, *Beyond Sixty-Five*. Also, see W. Achenbaum, "Obsolescence of Old Age in America, 1865–1914." For an account of similar trends in Germany, see Hans Joachim Von Kondratowitz, "The Medicalization of Old Age: Continuity and Change in Germany From the Late-Eighteenth-Century to the

Early Twentieth Century," in Pelling and Smith (eds.), *Life, Death and the Elderly*, 134–64, 138.

83 *AR* (1897), 211; and *AR* (1898), 151.

84 *AR* (1897), 4.

85 Haber, "And the Fear of the Poorhouse," 48.

CHAPTER 2

1 See Tamera Hareven, "The Last Stage: Historical Adulthood and Old Age," in *Aging, Death and the Completion of Being*, ed. David Van Tassel (Philadelphia, PA.: Temple University Press 1979); and Daniel Scott Smith, "A Community-based Sample of the Older Population from the 1880 and 1900 United States Manuscript Census," *Historical Methods*, vol. 2 (1978), 67–74.

2 Some studies tend to highlight more recent demographic changes and, as a result, though perhaps unintentionally, downplay changes that occurred before 1900. While these studies do not dismiss nineteenth-century developments, they do leave the reader with the impression that these were insignificant compared to later demographic alterations. See George Emery, "A Case-study Approach to Ontario Mortality History: The Example of Ingersol, 1881–1972," *Canadian Studies in Population*, vol. 15, no. 2 (1988): 135–58; and Kevin McQuillan, "Ontario Mortality Patterns, 1861–1921," *Canadian Studies in Population*, vol. 12, no. 1 (1985): 31–48.

3 See "Population by Age," in the printed volumes of the *Census of Canada* for the years 1851, 1891, and 1901.

4 See Richard Splane, *Social Welfare in Ontario, 1793–1893* (Toronto: University of Toronto Press, 1966), 106–7.

5 M.S. Marzouk, "Aging, Age Specific Health Care Costs and the Future Health Care Burden in Canada," *Canadian Public Policy*, vol. 17, no. 4 (1991): 490–506, 490. For information regarding the nineteenth-century decline in Ontario fertility rates, see Marvin McInnis, "Women, Work and Childbearing: Ontario in the Second Half of the Nineteenth-Century," *Histoire Sociale / Social History* (November 1991): 237–62, 238.

6 See "Population by Age," *Census of Canada* (1851, 1891, and 1901).

7 See John Demos, "Old Age in Early New England," in Van Tassel (ed.), *Aging, Death and Completion of Being*, 131.

8 See Ellen Gee, "Demographic Change and Inter-generational Relations in Canadian Families: Findings and Social Policy Implications," *Canadian Public Policy*, vol. 16, no. 2 (June 1990): 191–9.

9 As with the elderly portion of the population, it is difficult to compare with any precision the adult population of one period with that of another because of the way in which the age groupings in the census material changed over time. In 1851 and 1861 the adult population included all those over

the age of twenty, in 1871 all people over the age of twenty-one and in 1891 and 1901 all people over the age of nineteen.

10 David Troyansky, *Old Age in the Old Regime: Image and Experience in the Eighteenth-Century France* (London: Cornell University Press 1989), 10; David Thomson, "The Decline in Social Welfare: Falling State Support for the Elderly since Early Victorian Times," *Ageing and Society*, vol. 4, no. 4 (1984): 451–82; and David Thomson, "I Am Not My Father's Keeper: Families and the Elderly in Nineteenth-Century England," *Law and History Review*, vol. 2, no. 2 (fall 1984): 265–86.

11 Peter Laslett, "The History of Aging and the Aged," in *Family Life and Illicit Love in Earlier Generations: Essays in Historical Sociology* (Cambridge, U.K.: Cambridge University Press 1977), 187–9.

12 Lynne Marks, "Charity and Poor Relief in Late Nineteenth Century Small Town Ontario: The Mutability of Gender Roles and the Intersections of Public and Private" (paper presented at a joint session of the Canadian Historical Association and the Canadian Political Science Association, Ottawa, June 1993), 1. Marks points out that most social history in Ontario has focused on the urban experience, especially that of Toronto. In reality, however, the bulk of Ontario's people lived in small towns. Brockville was one such town.

13 See ibid.

14 See Peter Baskerville, "Mistaking the Census" (paper presented at the Demographic History Conference, University of Guelph, March 1993).

15 Brockville *Recorder* (1851).

16 For evidence of a similar trend in the United States, see Brian Gratton, *Urban Elders: Family, Work and Welfare Among Boston's Aged, 1890–1950* (Philadelphia, PA.: Temple University Press 1986), 27.

17 All information on Brockville's aged households, unless otherwise stated, was obtained from the manuscript census reports of Brockville for the years 1851, 1891, and 1901.

18 Ellen Gee, "Historical Change in the Family Life-Course of Canadian Men and Women," in *Aging in Canada*, ed. Victor Marshall (Markham, Ont.: Fitzhenry and Whiteside 1987): 265–87, 270.

19 Risa Barker and Ian Gentles, "Death in Victorian Toronto, 1850–99," *Urban History Review*, vol. 19, no. 1 (June 1990): 14–29, 14.

20 It is not possible to determine for certain if a wife listed in the census is a first or second wife. That a younger wife is a second wife is suggested in many cases by the presence of children in the household who are listed as the household head's offspring but who are obviously too old to have been the young wife's children. For instance, a thirty-five-year-old wife living with a sixty-two-year-old husband and his children, who are aged twenty-eight and twenty-four, is almost certainly not his first wife. Also, see Peter Ward, *Courtship, Love, and Marriage in Nineteenth-Century English Can-*

ada (Montreal: McGill-Queen's University Press 1990), 112. For evidence that old men married younger women specifically as a coping mechanism for old-age disability, see Margaret Pelling, "Old Age, Poverty and Disability in Early Modern Norwich: Work, Remarriage and other Expedients," in *Life, Death and the Elderly: Historical Perspectives*, ed. Margaret Pelling and Richard Smith (London: Routledge 1991): 74–101, 88–9.

21 These broad trends are comparable to what has been found by Michael Anderson in "Households, Families and Individuals: Some Preliminary Results from the National Sample from the 1851 Census of Great Britain," *Continuity and Change*, vol. 3, no. 3 (1988): 421–38. According to his findings, the portion of aged people who had adult children living with them in 1851 was lower (45 per cent) than was the case for Brockville. This, of course, is most likely a result of Britain having a more mature demographic structure at the time.

22 Ward, *Courtship, Love, and Marriage*, 181.

23 *Recorder*, 23 Dec. 1892, 6.

24 See Ruth Freeman and Patricia Klaus, "Blessed or Not? The New Spinster in England and the United States in the Late-Nineteenth and Early Twentieth Century," *Journal of Family History*, vol. 9, no. 4 (winter 1984): 394–414. Also, see Michael Anderson, "The Social Position of Spinsters in Mid-Victorian Britain," *Journal of Family History*, vol. 9, no. 4 (winter 1984): 377–93.

25 Gee, "Demographic Change and Inter-generational Relations," 195.

26 See Katherine McKenna, "Options for Elite Women in Early Upper Canadian Society: The Case of the Powell Family," in *Historical Essays on Upper Canada: New Perspectives*, ed. J.K. Johnson and Bruce Wilson (Ottawa: Carleton University Press 1991): 401–24, 404; Marvin McInnis, "Women, Work and Childbearing," 248. For an opposing view, see Jane Errington, "Single Pioneering Women in Upper Canada," *Families*, vol. 31, no. 1 (February 1992): 5–19.

27 Lucy Sprague Mitchell, cited in Emily Abel, *Who Cares for the Elderly? Public Policy and the Experience of Adult Daughters* (Philadelphia, PA.: Temple University Press 1991), 26.

28 See Errington, "Single Pioneering Women," 7. She comments that women often remained single because of expectations imposed upon them by their families; this idea is elaborated upon by Emily Abel, *Who Cares for the Elderly?* (see chapter 2, especially 38).

29 McInnis, "Women, Work and Childbearing," 254–6. Similar trends concerning increasing numbers of people remaining single and living with elderly parents are noted in R. Burr Litchfield, "Single People in the Nineteenth-Century City: A Comparative Perspective on Occupations and Living Situations," *Continuity and Change*, vol. 3, no. 1 (1988): 83–100, 98.

30 For more details on this trend, see Hareven, "The Last Stage."

31 In 1851 there were also a few single men who lived in hotels or inns.

32 Although a small number of household heads who lived with their children also lived with other relatives such as the household head's mother or sister, only 3.4 per cent of the households headed by an aged individual contained only relatives other than children. Less than 3 per cent of the aged household heads lived with non-kin and most of these were labourers or apprentices most likely employed by the household head.

33 AO, RG 22, Surrogate Court Records, GS–2–84 and 84 (MS 857–989–1005), Leeds and Grenville Counties (1891–1915).

34 This definition has been used as well by Howard Chudacoff and Tamera Hareven, "From Empty-Nest to Family Dissolution: Life-Course Transitions into Old Age," *Journal of Family History*, vol. 4, no. 1 (spring 1979): 69–82, 82.

35 In 1851 the specific relationship of a person to the household head is not recorded. Hence, a related person with the same last name as that of the household head is assumed to be a parent, while a related person with a different last name is taken to be an in-law. This assumption is supported by the fact that in 1901, when the precise relationship to the household head was recorded, the portion of aged people who were indeed parents or in-laws was not drastically different than the numbers calculated for 1851 based on these assumptions.

36 There were only four people who did not live with their children or in-laws. Two lived with other kin, one was a servant, and one was a lodger.

37 Ellen Gee, "Marriage in Nineteenth-Century Canada," *Canadian Review of Sociology and Anthropology*, vol. 19 (1982): 311–25, 317; Gee, "Historical Change in the Family Life Course," 271; McInnis, "Women, Work and Childbearing," 238.

38 Gee, "Historical Change in the Family Life Course," 275. Also, see Stewart Tolany and Avery Guest, "Childlessness in a Transitional Population: The United States at the Turn of the Century," *Journal of Family History*, vol. 7 (1982): 200–19.

39 See Barkin and Gentles, "Death in Victorian Toronto."; McInnis, "Women, Work and Childbearing," 238; and Jane Synge, "Work and Family Support Patterns of the Aged in the Early Twentieth-Century," in *Aging in Canada*, ed. Victor Marshall (Toronto: FitzRoy 1980), 135–44. Also, see Gee, "Historical Change in the Family Life Course," 275.

40 Chudacoff and Hareven, "From the Empty-Nest to Family Dissolution," 82.

CHAPTER 3

1 This trend has recently been reversed by the work of scholars such as Carole Haber and Brian Gratton. See their "Aging in America: The Perspective of History," in *Handbook of the Humanities and Aging*, ed. Thomas Cole,

David Van Tassel, and Robert Kastenbaum (New York: Springer 1992): 352–70. Other examples of their work are cited throughout this chapter.

2 Richard Deaton, *The Political Economy of Pensions: Power, Politics and Social Change in Canada, Great Britain and the United States* (Vancouver: University of British Columbia Press 1989), 17.

3 For example, see Sharon Cook, "A Quiet Place ... to Die: Ottawa's First Protestant Old Age Homes for Women and Men," *Ontario History,* vol. 81, no. 1 (March 1989): 25–41; James Snell, "Filial Responsibility Laws in Canada: A Historical Perspective," *Canadian Journal on Aging,* vol. 9 (1990): 268–77; James Snell, "The Gendered Construction of Elderly Marriage, 1900–1950," *Canadian Journal on Aging,* vol. 12, no. 4 (1993): 509–23; James Snell, "Maintenance Agreements for the Elderly: Canada, 1900–1951," *Journal,* Canadian Historical Association (1992): 197–206; Stormi Stewart, "The Elderly Poor in Rural Ontario: The Inmates of the Wellington County House of Industry, 1877–1907," *Journal,* Canadian Historical Association (1992): 217–34; James Struthers, "Regulating the Elderly: Old Age Pensions and the Formation of a Pension Bureaucracy in Ontario, 1929–1945," *Journal,* Canadian Historical Association (1992): 235–56; Jane Synge, "Work and Family Support Patterns of the Aged in the Early Twentieth Century," in *Aging in Canada,* ed. Victor Marshall (Toronto: Fitzroy Press 1980): 136–46; and, most recently, James Snell, *The Citizen's Wage: The State and the Elderly in Canada, 1900–1951* (Toronto: University of Toronto Press 1996).

4 James Struthers, *The Limits of Affluence: Welfare in Ontario, 1920–70* (Toronto: University of Toronto Press 1994), 51.

5 Edgar-André Montigny, "Historiography of Destitution: Canadian Historians and Old Age" (paper presented to the Canadian Historical Association Annual Meeting, St Catharines, June 1996), 16.

6 Ann Shola Orloff, *The Politics of Pensions: A Comparative Analysis of Britain, Canada and the United States, 1880–1940* (Madison, WIS.: University of Wisconsin Press 1993), 152.

7 Sara Arber and Jay Ginn, "The Invisibility of Age: Gender and Class in Later Life," *Sociological Review,* vol. 39, no. 2 (May 1991): 260–91, 260.

8 See Brian Gratton and Francis Rotondo, "Industrialization, The Family Economy and the Economic Status of the American Elderly," *Social Science History,* vol. 15 (1991): 337–62, 338; and Brian Gratton, *Urban Elders: Family, Work and Welfare Among Boston's Aged, 1980–1950* (Philadelphia, PA.: Temple University Press 1986), 98.

9 Orloff, *The Politics of Pensions,* 148.

10 See Laurel Thatcher Ulrich, *Good Wives: Image and Reality in the Lives of Women in Northern New England, 1650–1750* (New York: Knopf 1982), 37.

11 Judith Husbeck, *Old and Obsolete: Age Discrimination and the American Worker, 1860–1920* (New York: Garland Press 1989), 1.

12 Desmond Morton, *Working People: An Illustrated History of the Canadian Labour Movement* (Toronto: Deneau 1987), 6.

13 Michael Katz, *The People of Hamilton, Canada West: Family and Class in a Mid-Nineteenth-Century City* (Cambridge, Mass.: Harvard University Press 1975), 160–1.

14 James Struthers, "The Provincial Welfare State: Social Policy in Ontario," *Journal of Canadian Studies*, vol. 27, no. 1 (spring 1992): 136–46, 136–7.

15 David Scott Smith, "Old Age and the 'Great Transformation': A New England Case Study," in *Aging and the Elderly: Humanistic Perspectives in Gerontology*, ed. Stuart Spiker, Kathleen Woodward, and David Van Tassel (Atlantic Highlands, N.J.: Humanities Press 1978), 96.

16 Gratton, *Urban Elders*, 40.

17 Roger Ramson and Richard Sutch, "The Decline of Retirement in the Years Before Social Security: United States Retirement Patterns, 1870–1940," in *Issues in Contemporary Retirement*, ed. R.R. Campbell and E. Lazear (Stanford, CA: Hoover Institution Press 1988): 3–37, 3; and Roger Ramson and Richard Sutch, "The Labour of Older Americans: Retirement of Men On and Off the Job, 1870–1937," *Journal of Economic History*, vol. 46 (1986): 1–30, 5–6.

18 David Burley, *A Particular Condition in Life: Self-Employment and Social Mobility in Mid-Victorian Brantford, Ontario* (Montreal: McGill-Queen's University Press 1994), 166.

19 See Gordon Darrach, "Occupational Structure, Assessed Wealth and Homeowning During Toronto's Early Industrialization, 1861–1899," *Histoire Sociale / Social History*, vol. 32 (1983): 381–410, 398.

20 David and Rosemary Gagan, "Working Class Standards of Living in Late-Victorian Urban Ontario: A Review of the Miscellaneous Evidence on the Quality of Material Life," *Journal of the Canadian Historical Association* (1990): 171–93, 172.

21 Gratton and Rotondo, "Industrialization," 351.

22 Gagan and Gagan, "Working Class Standards of Living," 176.

23 Gordon Darrach, "Early Industrialization and Inequality in Toronto, 1861–99," *Labour / Le Travailleur*, vol. 11 (1983): 31–61, 41.

24 Terry Copp, *The Anatomy of Poverty: The Condition of the Working Class in Montreal, 1897–1929* (Toronto: McClelland and Stewart 1974), 33.

25 Livio Di Matteo and Peter George, "Canadian Wealth Inequality in the Late Nineteenth-Century: A Study of Wentworth County, Ontario, 1872–1902," *Canadian Historical Review*, vol. 73, no. 4 (December 1992): 453–83, 469.

26 Gagan and Gagan, "Working Class Standards of Living," 183.

27 Gratton and Rotundo, "Industrialization," 355; David Thomson suggests similar trends among the aged in England. See David Thomson, "The Welfare of the Elderly in the Past: A Family or Community Responsibility," in

Life, Death and the Elderly: Historical Perspectives, ed. Margaret Pelling and Richard Smith (London: Routledge 1991): 194–221, 206.

28 See Jane Synge, "Work and Family Support Patterns," 141.

29 Gagan and Gagan, "Working Class Standards of Living," 182.

30 Di Matteo and George, "Canadian Wealth Inequality," 470.

31 Katz, *The People of Hamilton*, 83.

32 See AO, RG 22, GS–2–84 and 85, Surrogate Court Records, Leeds and Grenville Counties (1891–1901); and AO, MS 857–988 to 1006, Surrogate Court Records, Leeds and Grenville Counties (1901–15).

33 See AO, RG 22, MS 857–994 (#3879), Surrogate Court Records, Leeds and Grenville Counties (1905).

34 AO, RG 22, GS–2–84 (#1956), Leeds and Grenville Counties (1892).

35 AO, RG 22, GS–2–85 (#2768), Leeds and Grenville Counties (1898).

36 Ibid. (#2666 and #3038), Leeds and Grenville Counties (1897 and 1900).

37 AO, RG 22, GS–2–84 and 85 (#1998 and 2615), Leeds and Grenville Counties (1892 and 1896).

38 For further evidence in support of this point, see Cheryl Elman, "Turn-of-the Century Dependence and Inter-dependence: Roles of Teens in the Family Economies of the Aged," *Journal of Family History*, vol. 18, no. 1 (winter 1993): 65–85.

39 AO, RG 22, GS–2–85 (#2978), Leeds and Grenville Counties (1899).

40 AO, MS 857–996 (#4055), Surrogate Court Records, Leeds and Grenville Counties (1907).

41 Gagan and Gagan, "Working Class Standards of Living," 190.

42 See Carole Haber, "From Senescence to Senility: The Transformation of Senile Old Age in the Nineteenth-Century," *Interdisciplinary Journal of Aging and Human Development*, vol. 19, no. 1 (1984–85), 44.

43 J.B. Wentworth, "The Glories of Old Age," in S.G. Lathrop, *Fifty Years and Beyond; or Gathered Gems for the Aged* (New York: F.H. Revell 1881), 109, cited in Thomas Cole, *The Journey of Life: A Cultural History of Aging in America* (Boston, Mass.: University Press 1992), 143.

44 Lydia Child, *Looking Towards Sunset* (Boston, Mass.: Ticknor and Fields 1866), 109, cited in Cole, *Journey of Life*, 149.

45 Ibid., 145.

46 AO, MU 2294: Osler Papers (Correspondence), Ellen Osler to William Osler, 15 Sept. 1886.

47 Ibid., Ellen Osler to Lizzie, 1 March 1888.

48 Ibid., Ellen Osler to Chattie, 1 Dec. 1887.

49 Ibid., Ellen Osler to William, January 1887.

50 Ibid., Ellen Osler to William, June 1896.

51 Ibid., Ellen Osler to Britton Bath, May 1899.

52 AO, MU 3913, Diaries of Wilmot Cumberland, January 1881.

53 AO, MU 3910, Diaries of Wilmot Cumberland, October-December 1893.

54 Ibid., March 1893.

55 AO, Biographical Scrapbook, vol. 1, 47 (1917).

56 Ibid., 524.

57 Ibid., 204.

58 AO, MS 409, Diaries of William Cochrane, September-December 1896.

59 Jill Quadagno, *Aging in Early Industrial Society: Work, Family and Social Policy in Nineteenth-Century England* (New York: Academic Press 1982), 173 and chapter 7.

60 Orloff, *Politics of Pensions*, 138.

61 See Barbara Rosenkrantz and Maris Vinovski, "The Invisible Lunatics: Old Age and Insanity in Mid-Nineteenth-Century Massachusetts," in Spiker, Woodward, and Van Tassel (eds.), *Aging and the Elderly*, 95–125, 95.

62 Gratton, *Urban Elders*, 126.

63 See David Thomson, "The Decline of Welfare: Falling State Support for the Elderly Since Early Victorian Times," *Ageing and Society*, vol. 4, no. 4 (1984): 451–82.

64 See David Thomson, "The Welfare of the Elderly in the Past," 217; and David Thomson, "The Decline of Social Welfare." Also, see Jill Quadagno, *Aging in Early Industrial Society*, 200.

65 See Sue Weiller, "Industrial Scrap-heap: Employment Patterns and Change for the Aged in the 1920's," *Social Science History*, vol. 13, no. 1 (spring 1989), 65–88, 66; Brian Gratton, "Labour-Force Participation of Older Men, 1890–1950," *Journal of Social History*, vol. 20 (1987): 689–710, 171; and Gratton, *Urban Elders* (introduction).

CHAPTER 4

1 See Susannah Moodie, *Roughing It in the Bush*, cited in David Murray, "The Cold Hand of Charity: The Court of Quarter Sessions and Relief in the Niagara District, 1828–1841," *Canadian Law in History Conference* (Ottawa: Carleton University Press 1987): 201–38, 201.

2 Alfred Kutzik, "American Social Provision for the Aged: An Historical Perspective," in *Ethnicity and Aging*, ed. Donald Gelfand and Alfred Kutzik (New York: Springer 1979), 33.

3 Laurel Thatcher Ulrich, *Good Wives: Images and Reality in the Lives of Women in Northern New England, 1650–1750* (New York: Knopf 1982), 9, 14. Also, see Laurel Thatcher Ulrich, *A Midwife's Tale: The Life of Martha Ballard, Based on Her Diary, 1785–1812* (New York: Vintage Books 1991); and Janet Finch, *Family Obligations and Social Change* (Cambridge, U.K.: Polity Press 1989), 101.

4 Ulrich, *Good Wives*, 14, 51.

5 Lynne Marks, "Charity and Poor Relief in Late Nineteenth-Century Small Town Ontario: The Mutability of Gender Roles and the Intersection of

Public and Private," (paper presented at a joint session of the Canadian Historical Association and the Canadian Political Science Association, Ottawa, June 1993), 7.

6 See Rainer Baehre, "Paupers and Poor Relief in Upper Canada," *Historical Papers*, Canadian Historical Association (1981): 57–80; and Murray, "The Cold Hand of Charity," 202.

7 Lynne Marks, "Charity and Poor Relief," 2. See also Ann Shola Orloff, *The Politics of Pensions: A Comparative Analysis of Britain, Canada and the United States, 1880–1940* (Madison, WIS.: University of Wisconsin Press 1993), 13.

8 See Adam Shortt and Arthur Doherty, *Documents Relating to the Constitutional History of Canada, 1759–1791* (Ottawa: Public Archives of Canada 1918), 943, cited in Richard Splane, *Social Welfare in Ontario: A Study of Public Welfare Administration* (Toronto: University of Toronto Press 1965), 66.

9 Margaret Kirkpatrick Strong, *Public Welfare Administration in Canada* (Chicago, Ill.: University of Chicago Press 1930), 119.

10 Murray, "The Cold Hand of Charity," 215. For evidence of similar sentiments in America during the same period, see Blanche Coll, "Public Assistance in the United States: Colonial Times to 1860," in *Comparative Developments in Social Welfare*, ed. E.W. Martin (London: George Allen and Unwin 1972), 128–58, 149.

11 Mary Stokes, "Local Government in the Shadow of the Law: The Municipal Corporation As Legal Actor in Canada West / Ontario, 1850–1870" unpublished paper, University of Western Ontario 1987, 4.

12 Kutzik, "American Social Provision for the Aged," 35; Coll, "Public Assistance in the United States," 145; Pat Thane, "The History of Provision for the Elderly to 1929," in *Ageing in Modern Society*, ed. Pat Thane (London: Croom Helm 1983), 192.

13 M.J. Heale, "Patterns of Benevolence: Charity and Morality in Rural and Urban New York, 1783–1830," *Societas*, vol. 3 (1973): 337–50.

14 Murray, "The Cold Hand of Charity," 214–19.

15 See John B. Williamson, Judith Shindal, and Linda Evans, *Aging and Public Policy: Social Control or Social Justice* (Springfield, Ill.: Charles Thomas 1985), 39; Ann Digby, *Pauper Palaces* (London: Routledge and Kegan Paul 1978), 161; and Orloff, *The Politics of Pensions*, 129.

16 See Margaret Pelling and Richard Smith, "Introduction," in *Life, Death and the Elderly: Historical Perspectives*, ed. Margaret Pelling and Richard Smith (London: Routledge 1992), 19. Also, see Lynne Hollen Lees, "The Survival of the Unfit: Welfare Policy and Family Maintenance in Nineteenth-Century London," in *The Uses of Charity: The Poor on Relief in the Nineteenth-Century Metropolis*, ed. Peter Mandler (Philadelphia, PA.: University of Pennsylvania Press 1990): 68–91, 87.

17 Thomas Wales, "Poverty, Poor Relief and the Life-Cycle: Some Evidence from Seventeenth-Century Norfolk," in *Land, Kinship and the Life-Cycle*, ed. Richard Smith (Cambridge, U.K.: Cambridge University Press 1984), 388; Elaine Clark, "Some Aspects of Social Security in Medieval England," *Journal of Family History*, vol. 7, no. 4 (winter 1982): 307–20, 316.

18 Murray, "The Cold Hand of Charity," 201.

19 James E. Smith, "Widowhood and Ageing in Traditional English Society," *Ageing and Society*, vol. 4, no. 4 (1984): 429–49, 438.

20 AO, RG 21, Municipal Records, F–1,566, Burford Township, Clerk Treasurers Records (1850).

21 David Roberts, "Dealing with the Poor in Victorian England," *Rice University Studies*, vol. 67 (1981): 57–74, 60.

22 Stokes, "Local Government in the Shadow of the Law," 8. On the similar situation in England and America, see E.W. Martin, "From Parish to Union: Poor Law Administration, 1601–1865," in *Comparative Developments in Social Welfare*, ed. E.W. Martin (London: George Allen and Unwin 1972), 25–56, 35; and Cray, *Paupers and Poor Relief*, 35–6.

23 See Stokes, "Local Government in the Shadow of the Law," 9, and Murray, "The Cold Hand of Charity."

24 AO, RG 22, Court Records, series 372, box 11, file 6 (Niagara District–Grand Jury Presentments, 1831).

25 Allan Irving, "The Master Principle of Administering Relief: Jeremy Bentham, Sir Francis Bond Head and the Establishment of the Principle of Less Eligibility in Upper Canada," *Canadian Review of Social Policy*, vol. 23 (1989): 13–18, 16.

26 Ibid., and Splane, *Social Welfare in Ontario*, 23.

27 Murray, "The Cold Hand of Charity," 204–5. See also David Thomson, "The Decline of Social Welfare: Falling State Support for the Elderly since Early Victorian Times," *Ageing and Society*, vol. 4, no. 4 (1984): 451–82.

28 AO, RG 22, series 372, Courts of the General Quarter Sessions of the Peace, Niagara District, box 36, file 16 (1839).

29 Murray, "The Cold Hand of Charity," 206.

30 Niagara *Mail*, 4 Oct. 1848.

31 Kenneth Bryden, *Old Age Pensions and Policy Making in Canada* (Montreal: McGill-Queen's University Press 1974), 34.

32 Since only a few petitions may exist from any given municipality or county, it is necessary to gather a variety of petitions from different locations and different decades to accumulate a sufficient number of examples to study. Nevertheless, no distinctions between the way petitions were dealt with were noticed.

33 AO, RG 21, F–1,628, East Gwillimbury Council Papers, box 3 (1859).

34 Ibid., series F–1566, Burford Township, Clerk Treasurer's Records (1850).

35 AO, RG 22, series 372, box 11, file 39, Court of the General Quarter Sessions, Niagara District (1832).

36 Perth *Courier*, 26 Feb. 1872.

37 AO, RG 21, Municipal Records, Raleigh Township, box 2, Petitions (1903).

38 Ibid., Raleigh Township, box 2, Petitions (1902).

39 Ibid., MS 178, reel 7, Town of Niagara Council Papers, 10 April 1868.

40 Ibid., Pittsburgh Township Petitions (1860), 25 June, Mrs Gordon.

41 AO, RG 22, series 37, Northumberland and Cobourg Petitions, box 1 (September 1823).

42 AO, RG 21: series F–1740, box 21: Leeds and Grenville County Council Papers, Petitions (1867).

43 This principal had existed in British communities since medieval times: see R.M. Smith, "Kin and Neighbours in a Thirteenth-Century Suffolk Community," *Journal of Family History*, vol. 4, no. 3 (fall 1979): 219–56, 219. It was also present in various nineteenth-century communities in Europe: see Peter Laslett, "Family, Kin and Collectivity as Systems of Support in Pre-industrial Europe: A Consideration of the Nuclear Hardship Hypothesis," *Continuity and Change*, vol. 3, no. 2 (1988): 153–75.

44 AO, RG 22, series 372, Court of the General Quarter Sessions of the Peace, Niagara District, box 8, file 5 (1832).

45 NAC, RG 5, Upper Canada Sundries: B 3, vol. 9, 1097.

46 Ibid., 1121.

47 AO, RG 21, series F–1740, box 23, Leeds and Grenville, Council Papers (1871).

48 Ibid., box 16, Leeds and Grenville Council Papers (Petitions)(1857).

49 Ibid., series F–1628, box 3, East Gwillimbury Council Papers (1878).

50 AO, RG 22, series 372, box 27, file 19, Court of the General Quarter Sessions of the Peace, Niagara District – Grand Jury Presentments (1837).

51 AO, RG 21, series F–1628, box 3, East Gwillimbury Council Papers, Petitions (1859).

52 See Michael Anderson, "Household Structure and the Industrial Revolution: Mid-Nineteenth-Century Preston in Comparative Perspective," in *Household and Family in Past Time*, ed. Peter Laslett (Cambridge, U.K.: Cambridge University Press 1972): 215–35, 231; and R.A. Parker, "An Historical Background to Residential Care," in *Residential Care: The Research Reviews*, vol. 2: 23.

53 Jill Quadagno, *Aging in Early Industrial Society: Work, Family and Social Policy in Nineteenth-Century England* (New York: Academic Press 1982), 88.

54 See Orloff, *Politics of Pensions*, 97; and Carolyn Rosenthol and James Gladstone, "Family Relationships and Support in Later Life," *Journal of Canadian Studies*, vol. 28, no. 1 (spring 1993): 122–38, 122.

55 See Christina Wolfson, Richard Handfield-Jones, *et al.*, "Adult Children's Perceptions of Their Responsibility to Provide Care for Dependent Elderly Parents," *Gerontologist*, vol. 33, no. 3 (June 1993): 315–23.

56 AO, MU 4563, Diaries of Anne McDonnell, 12 July to 31 Aug. 1805.

57 Agnes Hatfield, "Families As Caregivers: An Historical Perspective," in *Families of the Mentally Ill: Coping and Adaptation*, ed. Agnes Hatfield and H. Lefley (New York: Guilford Press 1987): 3–29, 4; and Emily Abel, *Who Cares for the Elderly? Public Policy and the Experience of Adult Daughters* (Philadelphia, PA.: Temple University Press 1991), 29.

58 For a detailed description of what duties housewives performed, see Ulrich, *A Midwife's Tale.*

59 Abel, *Who Cares for the Elderly?* 31. Also, see P.A. Pollett, I. Anderson, and D.W. Connor, "For Better or for Worse: The Experience of Caring for an Elderly Dementing Spouse," *Ageing and Society*, vol. 2 (1991): 443–69, 457.

60 See Abel, *Who Cares for the Elderly?* chapters 1, 2.

61 Brian Gratton, *Urban Elders: Family, Work, and Welfare Among Boston's Aged, 1890–1950* (Philadelphia, PA.: Temple University Press 1986), 52. Also, see Carole Haber and Brian Gratton, *Old Age and the Search for Security: An American Social History* (Bloomington, Ind.: University of Indiana Press 1994), 34; Tamera Hareven, "Recent Research on the History of the Family," in *Time, Family and Community: Perspectives on Family and Community History*, ed. Michael Drake (Cambridge, U.K.: Blackwell 1994), 13–43, 24.

62 Gratton, *Urban Elders*, 125.

63 Finch, *Family Obligations and Social Change*, 59.

64 Cheryl Krasnick Warsh, *Moments of Unreason: The Practice of Canadian Psychiatry and the Homewood Retreat, 1883–1923* (Montreal: McGill-Queen's University Press 1987), 71–3.

65 "Keep Up the Family Attachment," Perth *Courier*, 27 Sept. 1872. This point is important when one considers that it was usually only kin who lived nearby who cared for the aged. See Tamara Hareven, "Recent Research on the History of the Family," 24.

66 Orloff, *Politics of Pensions*, 3.

67 Ibid., 104. Also, see M.A. Crowther, "Family Responsibility and State Responsibility in Britain before the Welfare State," *Historical Journal*, vol. 25, no. 1 (1982): 131–45, 134.

68 Warsh, *Moments of Unreason*, 71–3; and Michael Katz, Michael Doucet, and Mark Stern, *The Social Organization of Early Industrial Capitalism* (Cambridge, Mass.: Harvard University Press 1982), chapter 3. See also Able, *Who Cares for the Elderly?* 78.

69 Similar findings were reported for England and Boston. See Quadagno, *Aging in Early Industrial Society*, and Gratton, *Urban Elders*.

70 Rosenthol and Gladstone, "Family Relationships and Support in Later Life," 122.

71 AO, Manuscripts on Microfilm, B-11, William Waind, "I Put it in My Memory: Reminiscences of William George Waind at Age 95," 38.

72 Ibid., 49.

73 AO, MU 757, Crawford Papers, box 4 (genealogical material).

74 See the Brockville *Recorder*, 17 Nov. 1899, and the Kingston *Whig*, 16 June 1898.

75 AO, MU 2294, Osler Papers, Ellen Osler to Chattie, 7 Sept. 1887.

76 AO, MU 3910, Correspondence Helen Pritchard to Wilmot Cumberland, 22 May 1893.

77 Janet Finch, "Do Families Support Each Other More or Less Than in the Past," in Michael Drake (ed.), *Time, Family and Community*, 96.

78 See Peter Laslett, "Family, Kinship and Collectivity As Systems of Support"; and Thomas Wales, "Poverty, Poor-Relief and the Life-Cycle," 383.

79 Richard Splane, *Social Welfare in Ontario*, 17; and Andrew Scull, "A Convenient Place to Get Rid of Inconvenient People: The Victorian Asylum," *Buildings and Society*, ed. A.D. King (London: Routledge and Kegan Paul 1980), 37–60, 38.

80 Cray, *Paupers and Poor Relief*, 199. Also, see Charles Lee, "Public Poor Relief and the Massachusetts Community, 1620–1715," *New England Quarterly*, vol. 55 (December 1982): 564–85; and Gary Nash, "Poverty and Poor Relief in Pre-revolutionary Philadelphia," *William and Mary Quarterly*, vol. 33 (January 1976): 3–30.

81 Virginia Burnhard, "Poverty and the Social Order in Seventeenth-Century Virginia," *Virginia Magazine of History and Biography*, vol. 85 (April 1977): 141–55, 148–9; David Schneider, "The Patchwork of Relief in Provincial New York," *Social Services Review*, vol. 12 (December 1938): 469–94, 465; Seamus Metress, "The History of Irish-American Care of the Aged," *Social Services Review*, vol. 59, no. 1 (March 1985): 18–31, 19. For a detailed image of how community support networks functioned, see Ulrich, *A Midwife's Tale*.

82 See J.B. Williamson, "Old Age Relief Policies Prior to 1900: The Trend Towards Restrictiveness," *American Journal of Economics and Sociology*, vol. 43, no. 3 (1984): 369–84, 371; and Priscilla F. Clement, *Welfare and the Poor in the Nineteenth-Century City: Philadelphia, 1800–1854* (London; Associated University Press 1985), 45; Joan Underhill Hannon, "Poor Relief in Antebellum New York State: The Rise and Decline of the Poorhouse," *Explorations in Economic History*, vol. 22 (1985): 233–56, 234.

83 Niagara *Mail*, 10 March 1847.

84 Perth *Courier*, 3 Jan. 1862, and AO, Mary Gapper O'Brien, Diaries, Journal, 28 Jan. 1830, 6.

85 AO, MU 843, Diaries Collection, Anne Patterson, 2 April 1881.

86 Ibid., Mary Gapper O'Brien, January 1830, 6.

87 Ibid., 9 May 1829, 14.

88 Ibid., February 1829.

89 Ibid., Journal, 1828, 4.

90 Jill Quadagno, *Aging in Early Industrial Society*, 123. See also Williamson, Shindul, and Evans, *Aging and Public Policy*, 39–40.

91 AO, RG 21, series F–1566, Burford Township, Clerk Treasurer's Records (1850).

92 AO, RG 22, series 372, box 9, file 12, Courts of the General Quarter Sessions of the Peace, Niagara District (1831).

93 AO, RG 21, Pittsburgh Township, Council Papers (June 1859).

94 AO, RG 22, series 372, box 25, file 17, Court of the General Quarter Sessions of the Peace, Niagara District.

95 Ibid.: series 37, Northumberland and Durham (1841).

96 AO, RG 21, F–1638, East Gwillimbury, Council Papers, box 3 (1860).

97 Ibid., MS 168, Western District Municipal Records (1846).

98 Ibid., MS 178, reel 5, Town of Niagara Council Papers (1852–8).

99 AO, RG 22, series F–1721, box 7, Court of the General Quarter Session of the Peace, Johnston District (1847).

100 Ibid. (1849).

101 AO, RG 21, series F–1740, box 18, file 1, Council Papers, Leeds and Grenville (1861).

102 AO, RG 22, series 372, box 33A, file 14, Courts of the General Quarter Sessions of the Peace, Niagara District (1839).

103 AO, RG 21, series F–1740, box 21, Leeds and Grenville, Council Papers (1860).

104 AO, RG 22, series 372, box 20, file 14, Court of the General Quarter Sessions of the Peace, Niagara District (1835).

105 AO, RG 21, F–1740, box 12, file 13, Leeds and Grenville County Council (1850).

106 AO, RG 22, series F–1,721, Courts of the General Quarter Sessions of the Peace, Johnston District, 1849.

107 AO, RG 21, series 372, box 11, Courts of the General Quarter Sessions of the Peace, Niagara District (1832).

CHAPTER 5

1 See Michael Katz, *In The Shadow of the Poorhouse: A Social History of Welfare in America* (New York: Basic Books 1986), introduction.

2 Priscilla Clement, *Welfare and the Poor in the Nineteenth-Century City: Philadelphia, 1800–1854* (London: Associated University Press 1985), 20–1.

3 See David Thomson, "The Welfare of the Elderly in the Past: A Family or Community Responsibility," in *Life, Death and the Elderly: Historical Perspectives*, ed. Margaret Pelling and Richard Smith (London: Routledge 1991), 194–221, 196; David Thomson, "Welfare and Historians," in *The World We Have Gained*, ed. L. Bonfield, R. Smith, and K. Wrightson (New York: Basil Blackwell 1986), 355–78, 365; and Janet Finch, *Family Obligations and Social Change* (Cambridge U.K.: Polity Press 1989), 11.

4 W. Newman-Brown "The Receipt of Poor Relief and the Family Situation in Aldenham, Hertfordshire, 1650–1690," in *Land, Kinship and the Life-Cycle*, ed. R. Smith (Cambridge U.K.: Cambridge University Press 1984), 420.

5 See E.H. Hunt, "Paupers and Pensioners: Past and Present," *Ageing and Society*, vol. 9, no. 4 (December 1989): 407–30. Even if Hunt's contention that Thomson exaggerated the generosity of nineteenth-century pensions is valid, Thomson's work still casts sufficient doubt upon traditional accounts of poor relief in the past to make his thesis worthy of further consideration; indeed, Thomson's thesis has been supported by recent research. For instance, benefits provided for lone-parent families appear to have followed the same pattern as Thomson described for public-support payments to the aged. See Keith Snell and J. Millar, "Lone-parent Families and the Welfare State: Past and Present," *Continuity and Change*, vol. 2 (1987), 387–422.

6 See David Thomson, "The Decline of Social Welfare: Falling State Support for the Elderly since Early Victorian Times," *Ageing and Society*, vol. 4, no. 4 (1984): 451–82 (chart on 453).

7 Richard Smith, "The Structured Dependency of the Elderly as a Recent Development: Some Sceptical Historical Thoughts," *Ageing and Society*, vol. 4, no. 4 (1984): 409–28, 422. See also David Thomson, "The Elderly in an Urban-Industrial Society: England 1750 to the Present," in *An Aging World: Dilemmas and Challenges for Law and Social Policy*, ed. John Eeklaar and David Pearl (London: Claredon Press 1989), 55–61.

8 David Thomson, "The Decline of Social Welfare," 468, and David Thomson, "I Am Not My Father's Keeper: Families and the Elderly in Nineteenth-Century England," *Law and History Review*, vol. 2, no. 2 (fall 1984): 265–86, 267.

9 Jill Quadagno, *Aging in Early Industrial Society: Work, Family and Social Policy in Nineteenth-Century England* (New York: Academic Press 1982), 123; David Thomson, "I Am Not My Father's Keeper," 273. See also T.C. Wales, "Poverty, Poor Relief and the Life-cycle: Some Evidence from Seventeenth-Century Norfolk," in Smith (ed.), *Land, Kinship and the Life-Cycle*, 383; Richard Smith, "The Structured Dependency of the Elderly," 422; Michael Anderson, "The Impact on the Family Relationships of the Elderly of Changes, since Victorian Times, in Governmental Income Maintenance," in *Family, Bureaucracy and the Elderly*, ed. Ethel Shanas and Marvin Sussman (Durham, N.C.: Duke University Press 1977), 36–59; Lynn Hollen Lees, "The Survival of the Unfit: Welfare Policies and Family Maintenance in Nineteenth-Century London," in *The Uses of Charity: The Poor on Relief in the Nineteenth-Century Metropolis*, ed. Peter Mandler (Philadelphia, PA.: University of Pennsylvania Press 1990), 68–91.

10 Thomson, "I Am Not My Father's Keeper," 265. Also, see M.A. Crowther, "Family Responsibility and Family Responsibility in Britain before the Welfare State," *Historical Journal*, vol. 25, no. 1 (1982): 131–45, 133.

11 Blanche Coll, "Public Assistance in the United States: Colonial Times to 1860," in *Comparative Developments in Social Welfare*, ed. E.W. Martin (London: George Allen and Unwin 1972), 128–58, 132.

12 Robert Cray, *Paupers and Poor Relief in New York City and Its Rural Environs, 1700–1830* (Philadelphia, PA.: Temple University Press 1988), 53; and Peter Laslett, "Family, Kinship and Collectivity As Systems of Support in Pre-industrial Europe: A Consideration of The Nuclear-Hardship Hypothesis," *Continuity and Change*, vol. 3, no. 2 (1988): 153–75, 168.

13 Thomson, "I Am Not My Father's Keeper," 265.

14 Ibid., 271.

15 Christopher Gordon, "Familial Support for the Elderly in the Past: The Case of London's Working Class in the Early 1930's," *Ageing and Society*, vol. 8, no. 3 (September 1988): 287–320, 310–14.

16 See Jean Robin, "Family Care of the Elderly in a Nineteenth-Century Devonshire Parish," *Ageing and Society*, vol. 4, no. 4 (1984): 505–16.

17 Michael Anderson, "The Social Position of Spinsters in Mid-Victorian Britain," *Journal of Family History*, vol. 9 (1984): 377–93, 393.

18 For example, see Michael Anderson, "Households, Families and Individuals: Some Preliminary Results from the National Sample from the 1851 Census of Great Britain," *Continuity and Change*, vol. 3, no. 3 (1988): 421–38; Daniel Scott Smith, "A Community-Based Sample of the Older Population". Also, see Quadagno, *Aging in Early Industrial Society*, 18.

19 Thomson, "I Am Not My Father's Keeper," 275, and Thomson, "The Decline of Social Welfare," 451–4.

20 Donna Thomas, *The Problem of the Aged Poor: Social Reform in Late-Victorian England* (Calgary: University of Alberta Press 1969), 21.

21 Thomson, "Decline of Social Welfare," 452.

22 Coll, "Public Assistance in the United States," 154.

23 Ibid., 134–8; John Alexander, "The Functions of Public Welfare in Late-Eighteenth-Century Philadelphia: Regulating the Poor?" in *Social Welfare or Social Control: Some Historical Reflections on Regulating the Poor*, ed. Walter Trattner (Knoxville, Tenn.: University of Tennessee 1983); and John Alexander, *Render Them Submissive: Responses to Poverty in Philadelphia, 1760–1800* (Amherst, Mass.: University of Massachusetts Press 1980), 26.

24 Virginia Burnhard, "Poverty and the Social Order," 151. See also Margaret Pelling, "Old Age, Poverty and Disability in Early Modern Norwich: Work, Remarriage and other Expedients," in Pelling and Smith (eds.), *Life, Death and the Elderly*, 74–101, 75; Ann Shola Orloff, *The Politics of Pensions: A*

Comparative Analysis of Britain, Canada and the United States, 1880–1940
(Madison, Wis.: University of Wisconsin Press 1993), 123.

25 Raymond Mohl, "The Abolition of Public Outdoor Relief, 1870–1900: A
Critique of the Piven and Cloward Thesis," in Trattner (ed.), *Social Welfare
or Social Control*, 35–50, 41.

26 Clement, *Welfare and the Poor*, 165.

27 Alexander, "Functions of Public Welfare," 25–7. Also, see Samuel Reznick,
"Patterns of Thought and Action in an American Depression, 1882–86,"
American Historical Review, vol. 61 (January 1956): 284–306; and Samuel
Reznick, "Unemployment, Unrest and Relief in the United States During
the Depression of 1893–97," *Journal of Political Economy*, vol. 61 (August
1953): 324–45.

28 Barry Kaplan, "Reformers and Charity: The Abolition of Public Outdoor
Relief in New York City, 1870–1898," *Social Sciences Review*, vol. 52 (June
1978): 202–14, 203.

29 Mohl, "The Abolition of Public Outdoor Relief," 41.

30 Clement, *Welfare and the Poor*, 38–9.

31 Thomson, "Historians and Welfare," 373; Orloff, *Politics of Pensions*, 122.

32 Quadagno, *Aging in Early Industrial Society*; Thomson, "I Am Not My Father's Keeper," 277–80.

33 Donna Thomas, *Problem of the Aged Poor*, 22.

34 See Quadagno, *Aging in Early Industrial Society*, 123; and Thomson, "I
Am Not My Father's Keeper," 277.

35 Smith, "The Structured Dependency of the Aged," 422; David Thomson,
"The Decline in Social Welfare," 454; Pat Thane, "The History of Provision for the Elderly to 1929," in *Ageing in Modern Society*, ed. D. Jerome
(London: Croom Helm 1983), 194; and Ann Shola Orloff, *Politics of Pensions*, 120.

36 Orloff, *Politics of Pensions*, 120.

37 Michael Anderson, "Impact on the Family Relationships of the Elderly,"
45, and Quadagno, *Aging in Early Industrial Society*, 123.

38 Andrew Schull, "A Convenient Place to Get Rid of Inconvenient People:
The Victorian Lunatic Asylum," in *Buildings and Society*, ed. A.D. King
(London: Routledge and Kegan Paul 1980), 37–60, 38.

39 Orloff, *Politics of Pensions*, 154.

40 See Bruce Bellingham, "Waifs and Strays: Child Abandonment, Foster Care
and Families in Mid-Nineteenth-Century New York City," in *The Uses of
Charity: The Poor on Relief in the Nineteenth-Century Metropolis*, ed. Peter Mandler (Philadelphia, PA.: University of Pennsylvania Press 1990),
123–60, 125.

41 See Eli Zaretsky, "The Place of the Family in the Origins of the Welfare
State," in *Rethinking the Family: Some Feminist Questions*, ed. B. Thorne
(New York: Longman 1982), 188–224, 197–200.

42 Philip Mandler, "Poverty and Charity in the Nineteenth-Century Metropolis: An Introduction," in Mandler (ed.), *Uses of Charity*, 1–37, 13.

43 Orloff, *Politics of Pensions*, 161, and Cray, *Paupers and Poor Relief*, 128.

44 Stephanie Coontz, *The Social Origins of Private Life* (New York: Verso Press 1991), 272–3.

45 Ibid., 272.

46 Zaretsky, "Place of the Family," 192.

47 Lorna McLean, " 'Single Again': Widow's Work in the Urban Family Economy, Ottawa, 1871," *Ontario History*, vol. 83, no. 2 (June 1991): 127–50, 27.

48 Allan Irving, "The Master Principle of Administering Relief: Jeremy Bentham, Sir Francis Bond Head and the Establishment of the Principle of Less Eligibility in Upper Canada," *Canadian Review of Social Policy*, vol. 23 (1989): 13–18, 16–17. Also, see Rainer Baehre, "Paupers and Poor Relief in Upper Canada," *Historical Papers, Canadian Historical Association* (1981), 79.

49 Ibid., 59.

50 See David Murray, "The Cold Hand of Charity: The Court of Quarter Sessions and Poor Relief in the Niagara District, 1828–1841," *Canadian Law in History Conference* (Carleton University, June 1987), 201–38. See also Ruth Bleasdale, "Class Conflict on the Canals of Upper Canada in the 1840's," *Labour / Le Travailleur*, vol. 7 (1981): 9–39, 14.

51 For evidence of a similar financial crisis in local poor relief in the United States, see Raymond Mohl, "Three Centuries of American Public Welfare, 1600–1932," *Current History*, vol. 65 (1973): 6–10, 8.

52 Richard Splane, *Social Welfare in Ontario, 1793–1893* (Toronto: University of Toronto Press 1965), 70.

53 See Joan Underhill Hannon, "Poor Relief in Antebellum New York State: The Rise and Decline of the Poorhouse," *Explorations in Economic History*, vol. 22 (1985): 233–56, 234.

54 Irving, "Master Principle in Administering Relief," 15–17.

55 For reference to this process in England and Europe, see J.S. Zainaldin and P.L. Tyor, "Asylums and Society: An Approach to Industrial Change," *Journal of Social History*, vol. 13 (1979–80): 23–48, 40.

56 Baeher, "Paupers and Poor Relief," 75.

57 Splane, *Social Welfare in Ontario*, 72.

58 Ibid., 74.

59 Elizabeth Wallace, "The Origin of the Social Welfare State in Canada, 1867–1900," *Canadian Journal of Economics and Political Science*, vol. 16 (1950): 383–93, 384. Also, see Philip Lee and A.C. Benjamin, "Intergovernmental Relations: Historical and Contemporary Perspectives," in *Fiscal Austerity and Aging: Shifting Governmental Responsibility for the Elderly*, ed. Carroll Estes and R. Newcomer (London: Sage Publications 1983), 59–83, 60.

60 Splane, *Social Welfare in Ontario*, 12.
61 Kenneth Bryden, *Old Age Pensions and Policy Making in Canada* (Montreal: McGill-Queen's University Press 1974), 22.
62 Splane, *Social Welfare in Ontario*, 109.
63 Ibid., 104. Also, see Carole Haber, *Beyond Sixty-Five: The Dilemma of Old Age in America's Past* (Cambridge, U.K.: Cambridge University Press 1983), 85.
64 CTA, SC 35, series H: "Report on Asylums and Hospitals," *Globe* 6 Feb. 1877.
65 Ibid.
66 Ibid., *Mail*, 22 Dec. 1876.
67 Ibid., "The Charity System," *Globe*, 24 Dec. 1879.
68 Ibid., series F: *Annual Report of the Toronto House of Industry* (1883), 4.
69 Stormi Stewart, "The Elderly Poor in Rural Ontario: Inmates of the Wellington County House of Industry, 1877–1907," *Journal of the Canadian Historical Association* (Charlottetown: 1992): 217–43, 224.
70 Andrew Schull, *Museums of Madness: The Social Organization of Insanity in Nineteenth-Century England* (London: A. Lane Publishers 1979), 40.
71 See Mary Stokes, "Local Government in the Shadow of the Law: The Municipal Corporation As Legal Actor in Canada West / Ontario, 1850–1870," (Unpublished paper, University of Western Ontario, 1987), especially 28–32 and n. 70. Also, see Mary Stokes, "Petitions to the Legislative Assembly of Ontario from Local Governments, 1867–77: A Case Study in Legislative Participation," *Law and History Review*, vol. 11, no. 1 (spring 1993): 145–80, especially 169, 176.
72 "Perth Municipal Council," Perth *Courier*, 31 Jan. 1862.
73 AO, RG 21, Municipal Records, Ontario County, Clippings Album.
74 Ibid., June 1878.
75 See ibid., Clippings Album; RG 21, series F–1886, Raleigh Township, House of Industry Reports; ibid., Lanark County, House of Industry Management Board Minutes; ibid., series F–1740, Leeds and Grenville (January 1893); and ibid., box 16, file 4, Leeds and Grenville (1857).
76 Ibid., series F–1740 (1883), file 111B, Leeds and Grenville.
77 "Ladies Aid Society," Brantford *Courier*, 19 Jan. 1887.
78 Splane, *Social Welfare in Ontario*, 109.
79 Ibid.
80 See Newmarket *Era*, March and April 1883; Brantford *Daily Courier*, 20 Dec. 1888. Note that in the fall of 1887 the Burford town council gave out $123, an average of $5 per person.
81 Perth *Courier*, 7 Jan. 1862.
82 AO, RG 21, Lincoln County Clerk Treasurer's Letterbook (see payments for destitute and insane).
83 Ibid., expenses for the Industrial Home (166, 466, 468).

84 Ibid., 1882–93, and House of Industry, Expense Book.
85 See various entries in the Brockville *Recorder* between 8 Dec. 1892 and 2 Feb. 1893.
86 This trend was discovered in Philadelphia by Carole Haber (*Beyond Sixty-Five*, 85) and in England by Tyor and Zainaldin ("Asylum and Society," 40).
87 Splane, *Social Welfare in Ontario*, 84.
88 CTA, SC 35, series H, *Globe*, 12 Oct. 1877.
89 David Thomson, "Workhouse to Nursing Home: Residential Care of Elderly People in England since 1845," *Ageing and Society*, vol. 3 (March 1983), 65.
90 See Anderson, "Impact on Family Relationships of the Elderly."
91 Quadagno, *Aging in Early Industrial Society*, 129.
92 Schull, "Convenient Place to Get Rid of Inconvenient People," 39. Also, see J.B. Williamson, "Old Age Relief Policies Prior to 1900: The Trend Towards Restrictiveness," *American Journal of Economics and Sociology*, vol. 43, no. 3 (1984): 369–84; and Benjamin Klenbaner, "Poverty and Relief in American Thought," *Social Services Review*, vol. 38 (1964): 382–99, 399.
93 AO, RG 21, Ontario County, Newsclippings Album (June 1877).
94 Ibid., Lincoln County – Clerk Treasurer's Letter Book.
95 Bryden, *Old Age Pensions and Policy Making in Canada*, 35.
96 Stewart, "Elderly Poor in Rural Ontario," 3.
97 Stephen Katz, "Alarmist Demographics: Power, Knowledge and the Elderly Population," *Journal of Aging Studies*, vol. 6, no. 3 (fall 1992): 203–25, 213.
98 Carole Haber, "The Old Folks at Home: The Development of Institutional Care for the Aged in Nineteenth-Century Philadelphia," *Pennsylvania Magazine of History and Biography*, vol. 110, no. 2 (April 1977): 240–57, 249. Also, see Haber, *Beyond Sixty-Five*, 126.
99 See *AR* (1891). Beds in institutions such as orphanages, lying-in hospitals, Magdalene asylums, schools for the deaf and blind, and reformatories were excluded from this total on the ground that they were highly unlikely to house older individuals.
100 *AR* (1897).
101 See *Ontario Sessional Papers*, no. 61 (1889).
102 See *AR*, "On Houses of Refuge for the Province of Ontario" (1896); and D.C. Park and J.D. Wood, "Poor Relief and the County House of Refuge System in Ontario, 1880–1911," *Journal of Historical Geography*, vol. 18, no. 4 (October 1992): 439–55, 446.
103 *AR* (1901).
104 Haber, *Beyond Sixty-Five*, 83.
105 Barbara Rosencrantz and Maris Vinovskis, "The Invisible Lunatics: Old Age and Insanity in Mid-Nineteenth Century Massachusetts," in *Aging and the Elderly: Humanistic Perspectives in Gerontology*, ed. Stuart Spiker,

Kathleen Woodward, and David Van Tassel (Atlantic Highlands, N.J.: Humanities Press 1978), 100–6.

106 Brian Gratton, *Urban Elders: Work, Family and Welfare among Boston's Aged, 1890–1950* (Philadelphia, PA.: Temple University Press 1986).

107 See Thomson, "Workhouse to Nursing Home."

108 CTA, SC 35, series H, "Provision for the Poor," *Globe*, 20 Oct. 1877.

109 Ibid., "Remodel it," *Evening Star*, 22 Sept. 1897.

110 AO, RG 21, series F–1740, no. 15, envelope 7, Leeds and Grenville (October 1853).

111 Ibid., series F–1551, Brant County, Correspondence (2 Jan. 1905).

112 For information concerning how this occurred in England, see Schull, *Museums of Madness*, 245.

113 Michael Meacher, *Taken for a Ride: Special Residential Homes for Confused Old People: A Study of Separatism in Social Policy* (London: Longman Group 1972), 2.

114 AO, RG 10, Inspector of Prisons, Asylums and Public Charities, series 20–F–1.

115 Gerald Grobb, "Explaining Old Age History: The Need for Empiricism," in *Old Age in a Bureaucratic Society*, ed. David Van Tassel and Peter Stearns (Westport, Conn.: Greenwood Press 1978), 42. Also see Gerald Grobb, *Mental Illness and American Society, 1875–1940* (Princeton, N.J.: Princeton University Press 1983), 181.

116 See Orloff, *Politics of Pensions*, 163–6. For an example of how this sentiment became embedded in relief practices, see Diane Matters, "Public Welfare Vancouver Style, 1910–20," *Journal of Canadian Studies*, vol. 14, no. 1 (spring 1979), 11.

117 Judith Husbeck, *Old and Obsolete: Age Discrimination and the American Worker, 1860–1920* (New York: Garland Press 1989), 170.

118 David Gagan and Rosemary Gagan, "Working Class Standards of Living in Late-Victorian Urban Ontario: A Review of the Miscellaneous Evidence on the Quality of Material Life," *Journal of the Canadian Historical Association* (1990): 117–93, 180.

119 *Ontario Sessional Papers*, no. 11 (1895), "27th Annual Report on the Common Gaol, Prisons and Reformatories," xii.

120 Michael Katz, *The People of Hamilton, Canada West: Family and Class in a Mid-Nineteenth-Century City* (Cambridge, Mass.: Harvard University Press 1975), 28.

121 Gregory Kealey and Brian Palmer, *Dreaming of What Might Be: The Knights of Labour in Ontario, 1880–1900* (Toronto: New Hogtown Press 1987), 206.

122 Ibid., 247.

123 See Marianna Valverde, *The Age of Light Soap and Water: Moral Reform in English Canada, 1885–1925* (Toronto: McClelland and Stewart 1991), introduction.

124 Allan Moscovitch and Glenn Drover, "Social Expenditures and the Welfare State: The Canadian Experience in Historical Perspective," in *The Benevolent State: The Growth of Welfare in Canada*, ed. Allan Moscovitch and Jim Albert (Toronto: Garamond Press 1987), 13–46, 18–19.
125 Stewart, "Elderly Poor in Rural Ontario," 17.
126 Michael Katz, *In the Shadow of the PoorHouse*, 88. Also, see Gratton, *Urban Elders*; Haber, *Beyond Sixty-Five*, 86; and Quadagno, *Aging in Early Industrial Society*.
127 Haber, *Beyond Sixty-Five*, 86, and Quadagno, *Aging in Early Industrial Society*, 132.
128 Ibid., 123.
129 McLean, "Single Again," 144.
130 Norman Patterson, "Canadian People, A Criticism," *Canadian Magazine*, vol. 12 (1899): 135.
131 *AR* (1895), 4.
132 *AR* (1899).
133 AO, RG 22, Court Records, series 372, box 24, file 15, Niagara District Court of the Quarter Sessions (Orders, July 1836). Also, see 26th *AR* (1893), 4.

CHAPTER 6

1 This term was coined by Andrew Scull. See Andrew Scull, "A Convenient Place to Get Rid of Inconvenient People: The Victorian Lunatic Asylum," in *Buildings and Society*, ed. A.D. King (London: Routledge 1980), 37–60.
2 *AR* (1899): (Hamilton), 126.
3 John Walton, "The Treatment of Pauper Lunatics in Victorian England: The Case of Lancaster Asylum, 1816–70," in *Madhouses, Mad Doctors and Madmen: The Social History of Psychiatry in the Victorian Era*, ed. Andrew Schull (Philadelphia, PA.: University of Pennsylvania Press 1981), 166–97, 189.
4 *AR* (1903): (Brockville), 129; and Barbara Rosencrantz and Maris Vinovskis, "The Invisible Lunatics: Old Age and Insanity in Mid-Nineteenth-Century Massachusetts," in *Aging and the Elderly: Humanistic Perspectives in Gerontology*, ed. Stuart Spiker, Kathleen Woodward, and David Van Tassel (Atlantic Highlands, N.J.: Humanities Press 1978), 116.
5 See Richard Fox, *So Far Disordered in Mind: Insanity in California, 1870–1930* (Los Angeles, Calif.: University of California Press 1978), 132.
6 *AR* (1896): (Mimico), 191.
7 Ibid. (1897): (Hamilton), 126. See also ibid. (1897): (Toronto), 3.
8 Thomas Brown, "Living with God's Afflicted: A History of the Provincial Lunatic Asylum at Toronto, 1838–1911," Phd Thesis, Queen's University, 1981, 24. Also, see *AR* (1893): (Toronto), 6.

9 *AR* (1896): (Hamilton), 127; and ibid. (1897): (Kingston), 94.

10 Ibid. (1899): (Hamilton).

11 Ibid. (1898): (Hamilton), 151.

12 Ibid. (1897): (Kingston), 93.

13 Ibid. (1903): (Brockville), 129.

14 See Gerald Grob, "Explaining Old Age History: The Need for Empiricism," in *Old Age in a Bureaucratic Society*, ed. David Van Tassel and Peter Stearns (Westport, Conn.: Greenwood Press 1986), 30–46, 42.

15 Andrew Scull, *Museums of Madness: The Social Organization of Insanity in Nineteenth-Century England* (London: Allan Lane Books 1979), 245.

16 Gerald Grob, "Rediscovering Asylums: The Unhistorical History of the Mental Hospital," in *Therapeutic Revolution: Essays in the Social History of American Medicine*, ed. Morris Vogel and Charles Rosenberg (Philadelphia, PA.: University of Pennsylvania Press 1979), 135–58, 147.

17 Grob, "Rediscovering Asylums," 147.

18 Scull, *Museums of Madness*, 253.

19 Ibid., 243.

20 *AR* (1903): (Brockville), 129.

21 Patricia O'Brien, *Out of Mind, Out of Sight: A History of the Waterford Hospital* (St John's: Waterford Hospital Corp. 1989), 139.

22 See *AR* (1898): (Brockville); ibid. (1897): (Brockville), 211; and ibid. (1897): (Toronto).

23 Ibid. (1862): (Rockwood, Kingston).

24 Between its opening and 1899 there were 2,754 patients treated, and all these case files are available. A further 1,405 people were treated at the asylum between 1900 and 1907. While the case files before 1900 are complete for both the male and female patients, after that date the male files are not complete. The female files after 1905 are incomplete as well. The actual number of cases can be determined from the annual reports of the asylum, but the case records for certain files cannot be located. For this reason, the totals used in the calculations that follow are based, not on the total number of cases treated at the asylum, but on the total number of case files located. However, the number of missing case files, especially files that pertain specifically to the aged, is small, and there is no reason to assume that the results of these calculations differ in any significant way from the figures that would have been obtained had the complete series of files been available.

25 *AR* (1899).

26 This number was obtained by examining the case files of the asylum. See AO, RG 10-20-F-1 (MS 717, reels 1–4). While some case files are missing, it is likely that if the missing files were to change the totals at all, the percentage would have been higher since the total percentage for the period prior to 1900 for which all case files were located was 9 per cent.

27 *AR* (1893): (Toronto), 1.

28 See Schull, "A Convenient Place to Get Rid of Inconvenient People."

29 Fox, *So Far Disordered in Mind*, 139.

30 All references to cases, unless otherwise stated, are from the microfilmed case files of the Rockwood Asylum for the Insane in Kingston, Ontario. These records are located at the AO in RG 10–20–F–1 (MS 717, reels 1-4). Access to them is restricted under the Freedom of Information Act. Under the stipulations of this act, only the first names of patients have been used and the case-file numbers have been omitted. To obtain the specific case-file numbers from the author, one must first fill in a Freedom of Information request form with the Archives of Ontario.

31 Peter Ward, *Love, Courtship and Marriage in Nineteenth-Century English Canada* (Montreal: McGill-Queen's University Press 1990), 51–2.

32 These figures are calculated using information from all case files for the entire period between 1866 and 1906. Owing to the small number of files in some periods, it is not possible to produce family-care statistics which would permit one to determine change over time. Only aggregate figures are possible.

33 Michael Meacher, *Taken for a Ride: Special Residential Homes for Confused Old People: A Study of Separatism in Social Policy* (London: Longman Group 1972), 2.

34 Walton, "The Treatment of Pauper Lunatics," 169.

35 See various case files from AO, RG 10, series 20–F–1.

36 John Walton, "Lunacy and the Industrial Revolution: A Study of Asylum Admissions in Lancashire, 1848–50," *Journal of Social History*, vol. 13 (1979–80): 1–22, 17.

37 John Walton, "Casting Out and Bringing Back in Victorian England: Pauper Lunatics, 1840–70," in *The Anatomy of Madness: Essays in the History of Psychiatry*, vol. 2, ed. W.F. Bynum, Roy Porter, and M. Shepherd (London: Tavistock 1985), 132–47, 135.

38 Brian Gratton, *Urban Elders: Family, Work and Welfare among Boston's Aged, 1890–1950* (Philadelphia, PA.: Temple University Press 1986), 153.

39 Emily Abel, *Who Cares for the Elderly? Public Policy and the Experiences of Adult Daughters* (Philadelphia, PA.: Temple University Press 1991), 31.

40 D. Hack Tuke, *The Insane in the United States and Canada* (Chicago, Ill.: Arno Press 1973; reprint of original 1885 publication). See report on Kingston Hospital.

41 Walton, "Casting Out and Bringing Back," 134.

42 Stephanie Coontz, *The Social Origins of Private Life: A History of American Families, 1600–1900* (New York: Verso Books 1991), 272–3; and Eli Zaretsky, "The Place of the Family in the Origins of the Welfare State," in *Rethinking the Family: Some Feminist Questions*, ed. B. Thorne (New York: Longman 1982), 188–224, 191–8.

43 *Report of the Medical Superintendent of the Toronto Asylum for the Insane, Journal of Legislative Assembly of the Province of Canada*, appendix 12, cited in Brown, "Living with God's Afflicted," 179.

44 Horatio Milo Pollock, *Family Care of Mental Patients* (New York: Arno Press 1976; reprint of 1936 original), 44.

45 Idris Williams, *Caring for the Elderly in the Community* (London: Chapman and Hall 1989), 219.

46 Fox, *So Far Disordered in Mind*, 97.

47 Agnes Hatfield, "Families As Caregivers: A Historical Perspective," in *Families and the Mentally Ill: Caring and Adaptation*, ed. Agnes Hatfield and H. Lefley (New York: Guilford Press 1987), 3–29, 4.

48 Fox, *So Far Disordered in Mind*, 11.

49 Meacher, *Taken for a Ride*, 2. Also, see RG 10, series 20-F-1.

50 See the *Report of the Medical Superintendent*. Also, see Fox, *So Far Disordered in Mind*, 44.

51 AR (1866).

52 Ibid.: (Toronto), 9. See also Wendy Mitchinson, "Gender and Insanity and Characteristics of the Insane: A Nineteenth-Century Case," *Bulletin Canadienne d'Histoire de Medicine / Canadian Bulletin of Medical History*, vol. 4, no. 2 (winter 1987): 97–117, 102.

53 AR (1882), "Report of the Medical Superintendent of the Rockwood Asylum, Kingston."

54 Charlotte MacKenzie, "Social Factors in the Admission, Discharge and Continuing Stay of Patients at Ticehurst Asylum, 1845–1917," in Bynum, Porter, and Shepherd (eds.) *Anatomy of Madness*, 147–74, 155. Mackenzie reports that the shame experienced by Victorian families when one of their members became mentally disturbed could be very intense.

55 Brown, "Living with God's Afflicted," 108.

56 AR (1899), 101.

57 See various files in R 10, series 20-F-1.

58 Meacher, *Taken for a Ride*, 40.

59 Lance Tibbles, "Medical and Legal Aspects of Competency as Affected by Old Age," in Spiker, Woodward, and Van Tassell (ed.) *Aging and the Elderly*, 127–52, 129. See also Williams, *Caring for the Elderly*, 219.

60 Ibid., 220.

61 Of all persons over the age of sixty admitted to Rockwood between 1858 and 1906, 52 per cent were described as uncontrollable, 40 per cent as dangerous or violent, and 22 per cent as suicidal. Seven per cent were listed as falling into of all three categories.

62 Walton, "Casting Out and Bringing Back," 141.

63 AR (1879), 351.

64 Grob, "Abuse in American Mental Hospitals in Historical Perspective: Myth and Reality," in *Sickness and Health in America: Readings in the His-*

tory of Medicine and Public Health, ed. Judith Leavitt and Ronald Numbers (Madison, Wis.: University of Wisconsin Press 1985), 298–313, 301.

65 Hatfield, "Families As Caregivers," 16.

66 Wendy Mitchinson, "Reasons for Committal to a Mid-Nineteenth-Century Insane Asylum: The Case of Toronto," in *Essays in the History of Canadian Medicine*, ed. Wendy Mitchinson and Janice Dickin McGinnis (Toronto: McClelland Stewart 1988), 88–109, 104–5.

67 Rosencrantz and Vinovkis, "The Invisible Lunatics," 120.

68 Cheryl Warsh, *Moments of Unreason* (Montreal: McGill-Queen's University Press 1989), 71–3.

69 See Hatfield, "Family As Caregivers," 5.

70 Walton, "Treatment of Pauper Lunatics," 189.

71 Brown, "Living with God's Afflicted," 276.

72 *AR* (1881), 375.

73 Fox, *So Far Disordered in Mind*, 46.

74 Walton, "Casting Out and Bringing Back," 141.

CHAPTER 7

1 James Struthers, *The Limits of Affluence: Welfare in Ontario, 1920–70* (Toronto: University of Toronto Press 1994), 55.

2 Ibid., 62.

3 For more details, see James Snell, "Filial Responsibility Laws in Canada: A Historical Perspective," *Canadian Journal on Aging*, vol. 9 (1990): 268–77.

4 Ann Shola Orloff, *The Politics of Pensions: A Comparative Analysis of Britain, Canada and the United States, 1880–1940* (Madison, Wis.: University of Wisconsin Press 1993), 120.

5 Ibid., 151.

6 For a detailed examination of how these pensions were administered in Ontario, see Struthers, *Limits of Affluence*, chapter 2, "Regulating the Elderly," 50–76. For more details concerning state support for the aged in Canada during this period, see James Snell, *The Citzen's Wage: The State and the Elderly in Canada, 1900–1951* (Toronto: University of Toronto Press 1996).

7 James Struthers, "A Nice Homelike Atmosphere": Aging and Long-Term Care in Post-World War II Ontario" (paper presented to the Second Carleton Conference on the History of the Family, Ottawa, May 1994), 4.

8 Ibid., 4.

9 Ibid., 10.

10 *Ontario Legislative Assembly Debates*, 33rd Legislature, 1st Session (1986).

11 Ibid., 30th legislature, 4th session, 477 (G. Sandeman, NDP, 14 April 1977).

12 Ibid., 32nd Legislature, 4th session, 1853 (R. Haggerty, Liberal, 20 June 1983); ibid., 33rd Legislature, 2nd session, 3656 (Hon. J. Sweeney, Liberal, 26 Nov. 1986).

13 Ibid., 35th Legislature, 2nd session, 3948 (Allan McLean, Progressive Conservative, 7 Dec. 1992).

14 For example, see ibid., 35th Legislature, 2nd session, 3959 (Elizabeth Witmer, Progressive Conservative, 7 Dec. 1992); *Partnerships in Long-Term Care: A New Way to Plan, Manage and Deliver Services and Community Support: An Implementation Plan* (Toronto: Ontario Ministry of Health 1993), 7.

15 *A New Agenda: Health and Social Services for Ontario's Seniors* (Toronto: Queen's Printer 1986), 1.

16 *Debates*, 31st Legislature, 2nd session, 4800–1 (David Warner, NDP, 9 Nov. 1978).

17 Ibid.

18 Ibid., 33rd Legislature, 2nd session, 987 (G.E. Morin, Liberal, 29 May 1986).

19 Ibid., 31st Legislature, 2nd session, 4803 (Hon. David Peterson, Liberal, 9 Nov. 1978).

20 Ibid., 31st Legislature, 2nd session, 4801 (M. Campbell, Liberal, 9 Nov. 1978).

21 Ibid., 33rd Legislature, 2nd session, Standing Committee on Social Development, s–788–93 (Hon. Ron Van Horne, Liberal, 20 Nov. 1986).

22 Ibid., 31st legislature, 4th session, 3435 (B. McCaffrey, Progressive Conservative, 16 Oct. 1980).

23 Ibid., 2860 (M. Bryden, NDP, 16 June 1980).

24 Ibid., 31st Legislature, 2nd session, 4801 (M. Campbell, Liberal, 9 Nov. 1978).

25 Bob Gardner, *Current Issues Paper #78: Community Support Services for the Elderly* (Toronto: Ontario Legislative Research Service 1988), 3.

26 *Debates*, 34th Legislature, 1st session, Standing Committee on Social Development, s–326 (Mavis Wilson, Liberal, 17 Nov. 1988).

27 Quoted in ibid., 31st Legislature, 4th session, 2827 (Frank Laughren, NDP, 13 June 1980).

28 Philip Resnick, "Neo-Conservativism and Beyond," in *Continuities and Discontinuities: The Political Economy of Social Welfare and Labour Market Policy in Canada*, ed. Andrew Johnson, Stephen McBride, and Patrick Smith (Toronto: University of Toronto Press 1994), 25–35, 26.

29 *Debates*, 33rd Legislature, 1st session, 1211 (David Warner, NDP, 29 May 1986).

30 Ibid., 1209 (David Warner, NDP, 29 Oct. 1985).

31 Ibid., 34th Legislature, 1st session, Standing Committee on Social Development, s–338 (M. Bryden, NDP, 17 Nov. 1988).

32 Ibid., 33rd Legislature, 1st Session, 1211 (David Warner, NDP, 29 Oct. 1985).

33 Ibid., 31st Legislature, 4th Session, 3439 (R. McClelland, NDP, 16 Oct. 1980); ibid., 34th Legislature, 4th session, 3948–50 (Allan McLean, Progressive Conservative, 7 Dec. 1992).

34 Ontario Nursing Home Association (hereafter ONHA), *The Ontario Nursing Home Association's Response to the Government's Redirection of Long-Term Care and Support Services in Ontario* (Markham, Ont.: 1992), 7, 16, and appendix 1–A.

35 This contention is supported by the research of Sheila Neysmith and Lillian Wells, who argue that for every person found in an institution there are two equally impaired elderly people living in private homes. See Sheila Neysmith and Lillian Wells, "Home Care: Who Defines the Priorities," in *An Aging Population: The Challenge for Community Action*, ed. Lillian Wells (Toronto: University of Toronto Press 1991), 96–107, 97.

36 ONHA, *Response*, 26, 38–9.

37 *Debates*, 35th Legislature, 2nd session, 1877 (Cameron Jackson, Progressive Conservative, 7 July 1992).

38 Ibid., 3950 (Allan McLean, Progressive Conservative, 7 Dec. 1992).

39 *Debates*, Standing Committee on Social Development, 34th Legislature, 1st session, S–395 (Bruce Owen, Liberal, 28 Nov. 1988).

40 Neysmith and Wells, "Home Care: Who Defines the Priorities," 105.

41 *Debates*, 35th Legislature, 2nd session, 3891 (Barbara Sullivan, Liberal, 3 Dec. 1992).

42 Ibid., 30th Legislature, 4th session, 481 (G. Sandeman, NDP, 14 April 1977).

43 *New Agenda*, 1.

44 Ibid., 34th Legislature, 2nd Session, 1011 (D. Cunningham, Liberal, 7 June 1989).

45 *Debates*, 34th Legislature, 1st session, Standing Committee on Social Development, S–395 (Mavis Wilson, Liberal, 28 Nov. 1988).

46 *Debates*, 35th Legislature, 1st session, 1649 (Steven Mahoney, Liberal, 3 June 1991).

47 Ibid., 34th Legislature, 1st session, 1007–8 (Hon. J. Sweeney, Liberal, 7 June 1989).

48 Government of Ontario, *Redirection of Long-Term Care and Support Services in Ontario: Questions and Answers* (Toronto: Queen's Printer 1994), 3.

49 *Debates*, 35th Legislature, 1st session, 1647 (Gary Malkowski, NDP, 3 June 1991).

50 ONHA, *Response*, 28.

51 Ibid., 4.

52 Allan Walker, "The Future of Long-Term Care in Canada: A British Perspective," *Canadian Journal on Aging*, vol. 14, no. 2 (summer 1995): 437–46, 443.

53 Senior Citizen's Consumer Alliance, *Consumer Report on Long-Term Care Reform* (Toronto: 1992), 15–18. See also Jane Leitch as quoted in *Debates*, 35th Legislature, 3rd session, 468 (C. Jackson, Progressive Conservative, 3 May 1993). Also: ibid., 35th Legislature, 4th session, 7033 (C. Jackson, 15 June 1994).

54 *Debates*, 35th Legislature, 3rd session, 464 (C. Jackson, Progressive Conservative, 3 May 1993).

55 Ibid., 474–5 (Hon. James Bradley, Liberal, 3 May 1993).

56 Ibid., 35th Legislature, 4th session, 7021 (Barbara Sullivan, Liberal, 15 June 1994).

57 Anne Bullock, "Community Care: Ideology and Lived Experience," in *Community Organization and the Canadian State*, ed. Roxana Ng, Gillian Walker, and Jacob Miller (Toronto: Garamond Press 1990), 65–82, 65.

58 Bullen, "Community Care," 76.

59 See Deber and Williams, "Policy, Payment and Participation," 296.

60 *Debates*, 35th Legislature, 3rd Session, Standing Committee on Social Development, s–1611 (C. Jackson, Progressive Conservative, 15 Aug. 1994).

61 Ibid., s–1616 (Geoff Quirt, 15 Aug. 1994).

62 Ibid., s–1609 (Barbara Sullivan, Liberal, 15 Aug. 1994).

63 Ibid., s–1610 (C. Jackson, Progressive Conservative, 15 Aug. 1994).

64 Community Care programs had begun in the late 1960s. It was not until 1976, however, that the government made explicit its commitment to such services. See Allan Walker, "Community Care and the Elderly in Great Britain: Theory and Practice," *International Journal of Health Services*, vol. 11, no. 4 (1981): 541–57, 546–7.

65 Margot Jefferys, "The Over Eighties in Britain: The Social Construction of Panic," *Journal of Public Health Policy*, vol. 4 (1983): 367–72, 369.

66 Janet Finch and D. Groves, "Community Care and the Family: A Case for Equal Opportunities?" *Journal of Social Policy*, vol. 9, no. 4 (1980): 487–514, 491; Bob Gardner, *Current Issues Paper # 78: Community Support Services for the Elderly* (Toronto: Ontario Legislative Research Service 1988), 20.

67 Jane Aronson, "Family Care of the Elderly: Underlying Assumptions and Their Consequences," *Canadian Journal on Aging*, vol. 4, no. 3 (1985): 115–25, 123.

68 Walker, "Community Care and the Elderly," 548.

69 Janet Finch, *Family Obligations and Social Change* (Cambridge, U.K.: Polity Press 1989), 128.

70 D. Challis and B. Davies, "Long-Term Care for the Elderly: The Community Care System," *British Journal of Social Work*, vol. 15 (1985): 563–79, 571; Finch, *Family Obligations and Social Change*, 129.

71 Finch and Groves, "Community Care and Family Care," 491.

CONCLUSION

1 See David Gagan and Rosemary Gagan, "Working Class Standards of Living in Late-Victorian Urban Ontario: A Review of the Miscellaneous Evidence on the Quality of Material Life," *Journal of the Canadian Historical Association* (1990): 173–93, 173–80.

2 Samuel Resnick, "Patterns of Thought and Action in an American Depression, 1882–86," *American Historical Review*, vol. 61 (January 1956): 284–306, 292. Also, see Samuel Resnick, "Unemployment, Unrest and Relief in the United States during the Depression of 1893–97," *Journal of Political Economy*, vol. 621 (August 1953): 324–45, 332; and Gaston Rimlinger. "Welfare Policy and Economic Development: A Comparative Historical Perspective," *Journal of Economic History*, vol. 26 (December 1964), 556.

3 *Ontario Legislative Assembly, Debates*, 34th Legislature, 1st Session, Standing Committee on Social Development, s–338 (M. Bryden, NDP, 17 Nov. 1988).

4 Bob Gardner, *Current Issues Paper #78: Community Support Services for the Elderly* (Toronto: Ontario Legislative Research Service 1988), 3.

5 *Debates*, 31st Legislature, 2nd Session, 4803 (Hon. David Peterson, Liberal, 9 Nov. 1978).

6 See Sheva Medjuck, Mary O'Brien, and Carol Tozer, "From Private Responsibility to Public Policy: Women and the Cost of Caregiving to Elderly Kin," *Atlantis*, vol. 17, no. 2 (spring-summer 1992): 44–58, 45; and see quote in Ellen Gee, "Demographic Change and Inter-Generational Relations in Canadian Families: Findings and Social Policy Implications," *Canadian Public Policy*, vol. 16, no. 2 (June 1990): 191–9, 195.

7 *Debates*, 35th Legislature, 3rd Session, Standing Committee on Social Development, s–1616 (Geoff Quirt, 15 Aug. 1994).

8 See AR (1863?) and Bruce Bellingham, "Waifs and Strays: Child Abandonment, Foster Care and Families in Mid-Nineteenth-Century New York," in *The Uses of Charity: The Poor on Relief in the Nineteenth-Century Metropolis*, ed. Peter Mandler (Philadelphia, PA.: University of Pennsylvania Press 1990), 123–60.

9 AR (1897: Brockville), 211.

10 *Debates*, 35th Legislature, 3rd Session, Standing Committee on Social Development, s–1611 (Cameron Jackson, Progressive Conservative, 15 Aug. 1994).

11 See Deber and Williams, "Policy, Payment and Participation," 315–16.

Bibliography

PRIMARY SOURCES

ARCHIVES OF ONTARIO
Manuscript Census Reports
  (1851) C–11734 Brockville
  (1871) C–10002 and C–10003 Brockville
  (1871) C–10000 Kingston
  (1871) T–6351 St Catharines
  (1891) T–6326–27 Brockville
  (1901) T–6460 Brockville
  (1901) T–6475–76 Kingston
  (1901) T–6480 St Catharines

Printed Census Reports
  (1851) Population by Age
  (1861) Population by Age
  (1871) Population by Age
  (1881) Population by Age
  (1891) Population by Age
  (1901) Population by Age

Collections
  L–8 Provincial Secretary, Printed Materials
  RG 10 Inspector of Prisons and Public Charities
  Series 20 Psychiatric Hospitals (Rockwood Asylum)
  Series 63 Printed Materials
  RG 21 Municipal Records
  RG 22 Court Records
  RG 22, GS–2–84, Surrogate Court Records: Leeds and Grenville Counties
  RG 63 Inspector of Prisons and Public Charities

Correspondence and Diaries
  Cochrane, William (1831–98) MS 409
  Crawford Family Papers MU 754–7
  Cumberland, Wilmot MU 3912–13
  O'Brien, Mary Gapper (1828–38) MS 199
  Osler Papers MU 2294, vol. 4 (Correspondence)
  Patterson, Alice (1862–68) MU 843, Diaries Collection

Manuscripts and Documents
  1841–67 Annual Report of the Board of Inspectors of Asylums and Prisons
  1867–1906 Report of the Inspector of Asylums, Prisons and Public Charities
  B 11 Wiand, William George. "I Put it in my Memory: Reminiscences of
  William George Waind at age 95."

Newspapers
  N1 Brantford *Courier*
  N144 Brockville *Recorder*
  N151 Kingston *Gazette*
  N Niagara *Mail*
  N276 Newmarket *Era*
  Perth *Courier*

CITY OF TORONTO ARCHIVES
SC 35, series F and H Toronto House of Industry

NATIONAL ARCHIVES OF CANADA
RG 5 Upper Canada Sundries
Ontario Legislature *Debates*

SECONDARY SOURCES

Abbot, Edith. "Poor Law Provision for Family Responsibility," *Social Services Review*, vol. 12, no. 4 (December 1938): 598-618.

Abbot, Grace. *From Relief to Social Security* (Chicago, Ill.: University of Chicago Press 1940).

Abel, Emily. *Who Cares for the Elderly? Public Policy and the Experiences of Adult Daughters* (Philadelphia, PA.: Temple University Press 1991).

Aber, Sara and Jay Gunn. "The Invisibility of Age: Gender and Class in Later Life," *Sociological Review*, vol. 39, no. 2 (May 1991): 260–91.

Aber, Sara. "In Sickness and in Health: Care-Giving, Gender and the Independence of Elderly People," in *Families and Households: Division and Change*. ed. C. Marsh and Sara Aber (London: Macmillian 1992), 86–105.

Achenbaum, W. Andrew. "The Obsolescence of Old Age in America, 1865–1914," *Journal of Social History*, vol. 8 (fall 1974): 48–62.

- *Old Age in the New Land* (Baltimore, Md.: Johns Hopkins University Press 1978).

Aitchinson, J.H. "The Development of Local Government in Upper Canada, 1783–1850," Phd thesis, University of Toronto, 1954.

Alexander, John. *Render Them Submissive: Responses to Poverty in Philadelphia 1760–1800* (Amherst, Mass.: University of Massachusetts Press 1980).

- "The Functions of Public Welfare in Late-Eighteenth-Century Philadelphia: Regulating the Poor," in *Social Welfare or Social Control? Some Historical Reflections on Regulating the Poor*, ed. Walter Trattner (Knoxville, Tenn.: University of Tennesse Press 1983), 15–35.

Anderson, Michael. "Household Structure and the Industrial Revolution: Mid-Nineteenth-Century Preston in Comparative Perspective," in *Household and Family in Past Time*, ed. Peter Laslett (Cambridge, U.K.: Cambridge University Press 1972), 215–35.

- "The Impact on the Family Relationships of the Elderly of Changes, since Victorian Times, in Governmental Income Maintenance," in *Family Bureaucracy and the Elderly*, ed. Ethel Shanas and Marvin Sussmen (Durham, N.C.: Duke University Press 1977), 36–59.

- "The Social Position of Spinsters in Mid-Victorian Britain," *Journal of Family History*, vol. 9 (1984): 377–93.

- "Households, Families and Individuals: Some Preliminary Results from the National Sample from the 1851 Census of Great Britain," *Continuity and Change*, vol. 3, no. 3 (1988): 421–38.

Angel, Jacqueline and Dennis Hogan. "The Demography of Minority Aging Populations," *Journal of Family History*, vol. 17, no. 1 (1992): 95–115.

Arber, Sara and Jay Ginn. "The Invisibility of Age: Gender and Class in Later Life," *Sociological Review*, vol. 39, no. 2 (May 1991): 260–91.

Arcury, Thomas. "Rural Elderly Household Life-Course Transitions, 1900–1980 Compared," *Journal of Family History*, vol. 11, no. 1 (1986): 55–76.

Aronson, Jane. "Family Care of the Elderly: Underlying Assumptions and Their Consequences," *Canadian Journal on Aging*, vol. 4 (1985): 115–25.

Baehre, Rainer. "Paupers and Poor Relief in Upper Canada," *Historical Papers*, Canadian Historical Association (1981): 57–80.

Ball, Ted. "Lobbying Government for Long-Term Care," in *Long-Term Care in an Aging Society: Choices and Challenges for the 90's*, ed. G. Larue and R. Bayly (New York: Golden Age Book 1992), 131–40.

Barkin, Risa and Ian Gentles. "Death in Victorian Toronto, 1850–1899," *Urban History Review*, vol. 19, no. 1 (June 1990): 14–29.

Bellingham, Bruce. "Institution and Family: An Alternative View of Nineteenth-Century Child Saving," *Social Problems*, vol. 33 (1986): 533–57.

- "Waifs and Strays: Child Abandonment, Foster Care, and Families in Mid-Nineteenth-Century New York," in *The Uses of Charity: The Poor on Relief in the Nineteenth-Century Metropolis*, ed. Peter Mandler (Philadelphia: University of Pennsylvania Press 1990): 123–60.

Benson, John. "Hawking and Peddling in Canada, 1867–1914," *Histoire Sociale / Social History*, vol. 28, no. 35 (May 1985): 75–83.

Binney, Elizabeth and Carol Estes, "The Retreat of the State and Its Transfer of Responsibility: The Intergenerational War," *International Journal of Health Services*, vol. 18 (1988): 83–96.

Binstock, Robert. "The Aged as Scapegoat," *Gerontologist*, vol. 23, no. 2 (1983): 136–43.

– "The Elderly in America: Their Economic Resources, Income Status and Costs," in *Aging and Public Policy: The Politics of Growing Old in America*, ed. W. Browne and Laura Katz Olsen (Westport, Conn.: Greenwood Press 1983): 3–34.

Bleasdale, Ruth. "Class Conflict on the Canals of Upper Canada in the 1840's," *Labour / Le Travailleur*, vol. 7 (1981): 9–39.

Bryden, Kenneth. *Old Age Pensions and Policy Making in Canada* (Montreal: McGill-Queen's University Press 1974).

Bullock, Anne. "Community Care: Ideology and Lived Experience," in *Community Organization and the Canadian State*, ed. Roxanna Ng, Gillian Walker, and Jacob Miller (Toronto: Garamond Press 1990): 65–82.

Burley, David. *A Particular Condition in Life: Self-Employment and Social Mobility in Mid-Victorian Brantford, Ontario* (Montreal: McGill-Queen's University Press 1994).

Burnhard, Virginia. "Poverty and the Social Order in Seventeenth-Century Virginia," *Virginia Magazine of History and Biography*, vol. 85 (April 1977): 141–55.

Bytheway, W.R. "Demographic Statistics and Old Age Ideology," *Ageing and Society*, vol. 1, no. 3 (November 1981): 347–64.

Chappell, Nena. *About Canada: The Aging of the Canadian Population* (Ottawa: Department of the Secretary of State of Canada 1990).

Child, Lydia. *Looking Towards Sunset* (Boston, Mass.: Ticknor and Fields 1866).

Chudacoff, Howard. *How Old Are You? Age Consciousness in American Culture* (Princeton, N.J.: Princeton University Press 1989).

Chudacoff, Howard and Tamera Hareven. *Transitions: The Family and the Life-Course in Historical Perspective* (New York: Academic Press 1978).

– "From the Empty-Nest to Family Dissolution: Life-Course Transitions into Old Age," *Journal of Family History*, vol. 4, no. 1 (spring 1979): 69–82.

Clark, Elaine. "Some Aspects of Social Security in Medieval England," *Journal of Family History*, vol. 7, no. 4 (winter 1982): 307–20.

Clement, Priscilla Ferguson. "Families and Foster Care: Philadelphia in the Late Nineteenth Century," *Social Service Review*, no. 53 (1979): 406–20.

– *Welfare and the Poor in the Nineteenth-Century City: Philadelphia, 1800–1854* (London: Associated University Press 1985).

Cole, Thomas. *The Journey of Life: A Cultural History of Aging in America* (Boston, Mass.: Cambridge University Press 1992).

Coll, Blanche, "Public Assistance in the United States: Colonial Times to 1860," in *Comparative Developments in Social Welfare*, ed. E.W. Martin (London: George Allen and Unwin 1972): 128–58.

Conrad, Christopher. "Old Age in the Modern and Post-Modern Western World," in *Handbook of the Humanities and Aging*, ed. Thomas Cole, David Van Tassel, and Robert Kasterbaum (New York: Springer Press 1992): 61–95.

Cook, Sharon. "A Quiet Place … to Die: Ottawa's First Protestant Old Age Homes for Women and Men," *Ontario History*, no. 81, no. 1 (March 1989): 25–41.

Coontz, Stephanie. *The Social Origins of Private Life: A History of American Families, 1600–1900* (New York: Verso Books 1988).

Cray, Robert Jr. *Paupers and Poor Relief in New York City and its Rural Environs, 1700–1830* (Philadelphia, PA.: Temple University Press 1988).

Crowther, M.A. "The Later Years of the Workhouse, 1890–1929," in *Origins of British Social Policy*, ed. Pat Thane (Totowa, N.J.: Rowman and Littlefield 1978): 36–55.

Dahlin, Michel. "Perspectives on the Family Life of the Elderly in 1900," *Gerontologist*, vol. 20, no. 1 (1980): 99–107.

Daniels, N. *Am I My Parents' Keeper? An Essay on Justice Between the Young and the Old* (New York: Oxford University Press 1988).

Darroch, Gordon. "Early Industrialization and Inequality in Toronto, 1861–1899," *Labour / Le Travailleur*, vol. 11 (1983): 31–61.

– "Occupational Structure, Assessed Wealth and Homeowning During Toronto's Early Industrialization, 1861–1899," *Histoire Sociale / Social History*, vol. 32 (1983): 381–410.

Deaton, Richard. *The Political Economy of Pensions: Power, Politics and Social Change in Canada, Britain and the United States* (Vancouver: University of British Columbia Press 1989).

Deber, Raisa and Paul Williams. "Policy, Payment and Participation: Long-Term Care Reform in Ontario," *Canadian Journal on Aging*, vol. 14 (1995): 294–318.

De La Cour, Lykke, Cecilia Morgan, and Marianna Valverde. "Gender Relation and State Formation in Nineteenth-Century Canada," in *Colonial Leviathan: State Formation in Mid-Nineteenth-Century Canada*, ed. Allan, Greer and Ian Radforth (Toronto: University of Toronto Press 1992): 163–91.

Demos, John. "Old Age in Early New England," in *Aging, Death and the Completion of Being*, ed. David Van Tassel (Philadelphia, PA.: University of Pennsylvania Press 1979): 115–64.

Denton, Frank and Byron Spencer. "Population Aging and the Future Health Care of the Elderly," *Canadian Public Policy*, vol. 9 (1983): 155–63.

Denton, Frank, C. Feaver and Byron Spencer. "Prospective Aging of the Population and Its Implications for the Labour Force and Government Expenditures," *Canadian Journal on Aging*, vol. 5, no. 2 (1986): 75–98.

Digby, Anne. *Pauper Palaces* (London: Routledge and Kegan Paul 1978).

Dilsworth-Anderson, Peggy. "Supporting Family Caregiving Through Adult Day-Care Services," in *Aging, Health and Family: Long-Term Care*, ed. T. Brubaker (Newbury Park, CA.: Sage Publications 1987).

Di Matteo, Livio and Peter George. "Canadian Wealth Inequality in the Late Nineteenth-Century: A Study of Wentworth County, Ontario, 1872–1902," *Canadian Historical Review*, vol. 73, no. 4 (December 1992): 453–83.

Easterlin, Richard, Christine MacDonald, and Diane Macunovich. "Retirement Prospects of the Baby-Boom Generation: A Different Perspective," *Gerontologist*, vol. 30, no. 6 (December 1990): 776–83.

Elman, Cheryl. "Turn-of-the-Century Dependence and Interdependence: Roles of Teens in Family Economies of the Aged," *Journal of Family History*, vol. 18, no. 1 (winter 1993): 65–85.

Emery, George. "Ontario's Civil Registration of Vital Statistics, 1869–1926: The Evolution of an Administrative System," *Canadian Historical Review*, vol. 64, no. 4 (1983): 494–518.

Emery, George and Kevin McQuillan. "A Case Study Approach to Ontario Mortality History: The Example of Ingersol, 1881–1972," *Canadian Studies in Population*, vol. 15, no. 2 (1988): 135–58.

Errington, Jane. "Single Pioneering Women in Upper Canada," *Families*, vol. 31, no. 1 (February 1992): 5–19.

Estes, Carroll, "The Reagan Legacy: Privatization, the Welfare State and Aging in the 1990's," in *The State, Labour Markets and the Future of Old Age Policy*, ed. John Myles and Jill Quadagno (Philadelphia, PA.: Temple University Press 1991): 59–83.

Estes, Carroll, Robert Newcomer *et al. Fiscal Austerity and Aging: Shifting Government Responsibility for the Elderly* (London: Sage Publications 1983).

Evans, Linda and John B. Williamson. "Social Security or Social Control?" *Generations*, vol. 6 (1981): 18–20.

Finch, Janet. *Family Obligations and Social Change* (Cambridge, U.K.: Polity Press 1989).

– "Do Families Support Each Other More or Less than in the Past," in *Family, Time and Community: Perspectives on Family and Community History*, ed. Michael Drake (Cambridge, U.K.: Blackwell 1994): 91–105.

Finch, Janet and D. Groves. "Community Care and the Family: A Case for Equal Opportunities?" *Journal of Social Policy*, vol. 9 (1980): 487–514.

Fischer, David Hacket. *Growing Old in America* (New York: Oxford University Press 1977).

Fox, Richard. *So Far Disordered in Mind: Insanity in California, 1870–1930* (Los Angeles, Calif.: University of California Press 1978).

Franke, James. "Support for Aging Policy: Self-Interest, Social Justice and Political Symbols," *Journal of Aging Studies*, vol. 1, no. 4 (winter 1987): 393–406.

Freeman, Ruth. "Blessed or Not? The New Spinster in England and the United States in the Late Nineteenth-Century and Early Twentieth-Century," *Journal of Family History*, vol. 9, no. 4 (winter 1984): 394–414.

Gagan, David. *Hopeful Travellers: Families, Land and Social Change in Mid-Victorian Peel County, Canada West* (Toronto: University of Toronto Press 1981).

Gagan, David and Rosemary Gagan, "Working Class Standards of Living in Late-Victorian Urban Ontario: A Review of the Miscellaneous Evidence on the Quality of Material Life," *Journal of the Canadian Historical Association* (1990): 171–93.

Gailleur, Xavier. "Economic Crisis and Old Age," *Ageing and Society*, vol. 2, no. 2 (1982): 165–82.

Gee, Ellen. "Marriage in Nineteenth-Century Canada," *Canadian Review of Sociology and Anthropology*, vol. 19 (1982): 311–25.

– "Historical Change in the Family Life-Course of Canadian Men and Women," in *Aging in Canada*, ed. Victor Marshall (Markham, Ont.: Fitzhenry and Whiteside 1987): 265–87.

– "Demographic Change and Intergenerational Relations in Canadian Families: Findings and Social Policy Implications," *Canadian Public Policy*, vol. 16, no. 2 (June 1990): 191–9.

Gee, Ellen and Susan McDaniel. "Social Policy for an Aging Society," *Journal of Canadian Studies*, vol. 28, no. 1 (spring 1993): 139–52.

Gilbert, Bentley. "The Decay of Nineteenth-Century Provident Institutions and the Coming of Old Age Pensions in Great Britain," *Economic History Review*, vol. 17 (1964): 551–63.

Gold, J.G. and S. Kaufman. "Development of Care of Elderly: Tracing the History of Institutional Facilities," *Gerontologist*, vol. 10, no. 4 (1970): 262–74.

Gordon, Christopher. "Familial Support for the Elderly in the Past: The Case of London's Working Class in the 1930's," *Ageing and Society*, vol. 8, no. 3 (September 1988): 287–320.

Gordon, Linda. "Social Insurance and Public Assistance: The Influence of Gender in Welfare Thought in the United States, 1890–1935," *American Historical Review*, vol. 97, no. 1 (February 1992): 19–54.

Graebner, William. *A History of Retirement: The Meaning and Function of an American Institution, 1885–1978* (New Haven, Conn.: Yale University Press 1980).

– "A Comment: The Social Security Crisis in Perspective," in *Old Age in a Bureaucratic Society: The Elderly, the Experts and American Historians*, ed.

David Van Tassel and Peter Stearns (Westport, Conn.: Greenwood Press 1986): 217–21.

Gratton, Brian. "The New History of the Aged: A Critique," in *Old Age in a Bureaucratic Society: The Elderly, The Experts and the State in American History*, ed. David Van Tassel and Peter Stearns (Westport, Conn.: Greenwood Press 1986): 3–29.

– *Urban Elders: Family, Work and Welfare Among Boston's Aged, 1890-1950* (Philadelphia, PA.: Temple University Press 1986).

– "The Labour-Force Participation of Older Men, 1890–1950," *Journal of Social History*, vol. 20 (1987): 689–710.

– "The New Welfare State: Security and Retirement in 1950," *Social Science History*, vol. 12, no. 2 (summer 1988): 171–96.

Gratton, Brian and F. Rotondo. "Industrialization, the Family Economy and the Economic Status of the American Elderly," *Social Science History*, vol. 15 (1991): 337–62.

Grob, Gerald. "Rediscovering Asylums: The Unhistorical History of the Mental Hospital," in *The Therapeutic Revolution: Essays in the Social History of American Medicine*, ed. Morris Vogel and Charles Rosenberg (Philadelphia, PA.: University of Pennsylvania Press 1979): 135–58.

– "Abuse in American Mental Hospitals in Historical Perspective: Myth and Reality," in *Sickness and Health in America: Readings in the History of Medicine and Public Health*, ed. Judith Leavit and R. Numbers (Madison, Wis.: University of Wisconsin Press 1985): 298–310.

– "Explaining Old Age History: The Need for Empiricism," in *Old Age in a Bureaucratic State: The Elderly, The Experts and the State in American History*, ed. David Van Tassel and Peter Stearns (Westport, Conn.: Greenwood Press 1986).

Haber, Carole. "The Old Folks Home: The Development of Institutional Care for the Aged in Nineteenth-Century Philadelphia," *Pennsylvania Magazine of History and Biography*, vol. 110, no. 2 (April 1977): 240–57.

– "Mandatory Retirement in Nineteenth-Century America: The Conceptual Basis for a New Work Cycle," *Journal of Social History*, vol. 12 (fall 1978): 77–96.

– *Beyond Sixty-Five: The Dilemma of Old Age in America's Past* (Cambridge, U.K.: Cambridge University Press 1983).

– "From Senescence to Senility: The Transformation of Senile Old Age in the Nineteenth-Century," *Interdisciplinary Journal of Aging and Human Development*, vol. 19, no. 1 (1984–85): 47–54.

– " 'And the Fear of the Poorhouse': Perceptions of Old Age Impoverishment in Early Twentieth Century America," *Generations*, vol. 17, no. 2 (spring-summer 1993): 46–50.

Haber, Carole and Brian Gratton. "Aging in America: The Perspective of History," in *Handbook of the Humanities and Aging*, ed. Thomas Cole,

David Van Tassel, and Robert Kastenbaum (New York: Springer Press 1992): 352–70.

– *Old Age and the Search for Security: An American Social History* (Bloomington, Ind.: Indiana University Press 1994).

Hannon, Joan Underhill. "The Generosity of Antebellum Poor Relief," *Journal of Economic History*, vol. 44 (1984): 810–21.

– "Poverty in the Antebellum North East," *Journal of Economic History*, vol. 44 (1984): 1,007–32.

– "Poor Relief in Antebellum New York State: The Rise and Fall of the Poorhouse," *Explorations in Economic History*, vol. 22 (1985): 233–56.

Hareven, Tamera. "An Ambiguous Alliance: Some Aspects of American Influence on Canadian Social Welfare," *Histoire Sociale / Social History*, vol. 3 (1969): 82–98.

– "The Last Stage: Historical Adulthood and Old Age," in *Aging, Death and the Completion of Being*, ed. David Van Tassel (Philadelphia, PA.: University of Pennsylvania Press 1979): 165–92.

– "The Dynamics of Kin in an Industrial Community," in *Families and Work*, ed. N. Gerstel and H. Gross (Philadelphia: Temple University Press 1987): 55–83.

– "Recent Research on the History of the Family," in *Time, Family and Community: Perspectives on Family and Community History*, ed. Michael Drake (Cambridge, U.K.: Blackwell 1994): 13–43.

Hatfield, Agnes. "Families As Caregivers: A Historical Perspective," in *Families of the Mentally Ill: Caring and Adaptation*, ed. Agnes Hatfield and H. Lefley (New York: Guilford Press 1987): 3–29.

Heale, M.J. "Patterns of Benevolence: Charity and Morality in Rural and Urban New York, 1783–1830," *Societas*, vol. 3 (1973): 337–50.

Hertzman, Clyde and Michael Hayes. "Will the Elderly Really Bankrupt us With Increased Health Care Costs?" *Canadian Journal of Public Health*, vol. 76 (1985): 373–7.

Himmelfarb, Gertrude. *Poverty and Compassion: The Moral Imagination of the Late Victorians* (New York: Random House 1991).

Hudson, R.B. "The Greying of the Federal Budget and Its Consequences for Old Age Policy," *Gerontologist*, vol. 18 (1978): 428–40.

Hunt, E.H. "Paupers and Pensioners: Past and Present," *Ageing and Society*, vol. 9, no. 4 (December 1989): 407–30.

Husbeck, Judith. *Old and Obsolete: Age Discrimination and the American Worker, 1860–1920* (New York: Garland Press 1989).

Irving, Allan. "The Master Principle of Administrating Relief: Jeremy Bentham, Sir Francis Bond Head and the Establishment of the Principle of Less Eligibility in Upper Canada," *Canadian Review of Social Policy*, vol. 23 (1989): 13–18.

Jan van der Veen, Willem and Frans Von Poppel. "Institutional Care for the Elderly in the Nineteenth Century: Old People in the Hague and Institutions," *Ageing and Society*, vol. 12, no. 2 (June 1992): 185–212.

Jefferies, Margot. "The Over-Eighties in Britain: The Social Construction of Panic," *Journal of Public Health Policy*, vol. 4 (1983): 367–72.

Johnson, Paul and Jane Falkingham. *Ageing and Economic Welfare* (London: Sage Publications 1992).

Kane, Rosalie and Robert Kane. "Home and Community-Based Care in Canada," in *Financing Home Care: Improving Protection for the Disabled Elderly*, ed. Diane Rowland and Barbara Lyons (Baltimore, Md.: 1991).

Kaplan, Barry. "Reformers and Charity: The Abolition of Public Outdoor Relief in New York City, 1870–1898," *Social Science Review*, vol. 52 (June 1978): 202–14.

Katz, Michael. *The People of Hamilton, Canada West: Family and Class in a Mid-Nineteenth-Century City* (Cambridge, Mass.: Harvard University Press 1975).

– *Poverty and Policy in American History* (New York: Academic Press 1983).

– *In the Shadow of the Poorhouse: A Social History of Welfare in America* (New York: Basic Books 1986).

– *The Undeserving Poor: From the War on Poverty to the War on Welfare* (New York: Pantheon 1989).

Katz, Stephen. "Alarmist Demography: Power, Knowledge, and the Elderly Population," *Journal of Aging Studies*, vol. 6, no. 3 (fall 1992): 203–25.

Kealey, Gregory and Brian Palmer. *Dreaming of What Might Be: The Knights of Labour in Ontario, 1880–1900* (Toronto: New Hogtown Press 1987).

Kearl, M.C., K. Moore, and J.S. Osberg. "Political Implications of the New Ageism," *International Journal of Aging and Human Development*, vol. 15, no. 3 (1982): 167–83.

Klebaner, Benjamin. "Poverty and Relief in America Thought, 1815–61," *Social Services Review*, vol. 38 (1964): 382–99.

Krasnick, Cheryl. "In Charge of the Loons: A Portrait of the London, Ontario Asylum for the Insane in the Nineteenth-Century," *Ontario History*, vol. 74 no. 3 (September 1982): 138–84.

Kutzik, Alfred. "American Social Provision for the Aged: An Historical Perspective," in *Ethnicity and Aging*, ed. Donald Gelfand and Alfred Kutzik (New York: Springer Publications 1979): 32–64.

Laslett, Peter. "The History of Aging and the Aged," in *Family Life and Illicit Love in Earlier Generations: Essays in Historical Sociology* (Cambridge, U.K.: Cambridge University Press 1977): 174–213.

– "The Traditional English Family and the Aged in Our Society," in *Aging, Death and the Completion of Being*, ed. David Van Tassel (Philadelphia, PA.: University of Pennsylvania Press 1979): 97–114.

– "The Significance of the Past in the Study of Ageing," *Ageing and Society*, vol. 4, no. 4 (1984): 379–89.

– "Family, Kinship and Collectivity As Systems of Support in Pre-industrial Europe: A Consideration of the Nuclear Hardship Hypothesis," *Continuity and Change*, vol. 3, no. 2 (1988): 153–75.

Lee, Charles. "Public Poor Relief and the Massachusetts Community, 1620–1715," *New England Quarterly*, vol. 55 (December 1982): 564–85.

Lee, Philip and R.E. Benjamin. "Intergovernmental Relations: Historical and Contemporary Perspectives," in *Fiscal Austerity and Aging: Shifting Governmental Responsibility for the Elderly*, ed. Carroll Estes, Robert Newcomer *et al.* (London: Sage Publications 1983): 59–83.

Lees, Lynn Hollen. "The Survival of the Unfit: Welfare Policies and Family Maintenance in Nineteenth-Century London," in *The Uses of Charity: The Poor on Relief in the Nineteenth-Century Metropolis*, ed. Peter Mandler (Philadelphia, Penn.: University of Pennsylvania Press 1990): 68–91.

Litchfield, R. Burr. "Single People in the Nineteenth-Century City: A Comparative Perspective on Occupations and Living Situations," *Continuity and Change*, vol. 3, no. 1 (1988): 83–100.

Livi-Bacci, Massimo. "Social and Biological Aging: Contradictions of Development," *Population and Development Review*, vol. 8, no. 4 (December 1982): 771–82.

Longman, Philip. *Born to Pay: The New Politics of Aging in America* (Boston, Mass.: Houghton Mifflin 1987).

Mandler, Peter. "Poverty and Charity in the Nineteenth-Century Metropolis: An Introduction," in *The Uses of Charity: The Poor on Relief in the Nineteenth Century Metropolis*, ed. Peter Mandler (Philadelphia, Penn.: University of Pennsylvania 1990): 1–37.

Marcel-Gratton, Nicole and Jacques Legaré. "Being Old Today and Tomorrow: A Different Proposition," *Canadian Studies in Population*, vol. 14, no. 2 (1987): 237–41.

Martin, E.W. "From Parish to Union: Poor Law Administration 1601–1865," in *Comparative Developments in Social Welfare*, ed. E.W. Martin (London: Geroge Allan and Unwin 1972): 25–56.

McCord, Norman. "Ratepayers and Social Policy," in *The Origins of British Social Policy*, ed. Pat Thane (London: Croom Helm 1978): 21–35.

McDaniel, Susan. "Demographic Aging as a Guiding Paradigm in Canada's Welfare State," *Canadian Public Policy*, vol. 13, no. 3 (1987): 330–6.

McInnis, Marvin. "Women, Work and Childbearing: Ontario in the Second Half of the Nineteenth-Century," *Histoire Sociale / Social History*, vol. 24 (November 1991): 237–62.

MacIntyre, Sheila. "Old Age As a Social Problem: Historical Notes on the English Experience," in *Health Care and Health Knowledge*, ed. R. Dingwall, C. Heath, and M. Reid (London: Croom Helm 1977): 41–63.

McKenna, Katherine. "Options for Elite Women in Early Upper Canadian Society: The Case of the Powell Family," in *Historical Essays on Upper Canada: New Perspectives* (Ottawa: Carleton University Press 1991): 401–24.

McLean, Lorna. "Single Again: Widow's Work in the Urban Family Economy, Ottawa, 1871," *Ontario History*, vol. 83, no. 2 (1991): 127–50.

McQuillan, Kevin. "Ontario Mortality Patterns, 1861–1921," *Canadian Studies in Population*, vol. 12, no. 1 (1985): 31–48.

Marks, Lynne. "Charity and Poor Relief in Late-Nineteenth-Century Small Town Ontario: The Mutability of Gender Roles and the Intersection of Public and Private" (paper presented at a joint session of the Canadian Historical Association and the Canadian Political Science Association, Ottawa, June 1993).

Marshall, Victor. "A Critique of Canadian Aging and Health Policy," *Journal of Canadian Studies*, vol. 28, no. 1 (spring 1993): 153–65.

Marzouk, M.S. "Aging, Age Specific Health Care Costs and the Future Health Care Burden in Canada," *Canadian Public Policy*, vol. 17, no. 4 (1991): 490–506.

Matters, Diane. "Public Welfare Vancouver Style, 1910–1920," *Journal of Canadian Studies*, vol. 14, no. 1 (spring 1979): 3–15.

Meacher, Michael. *Taken for a Ride: Special Residential Homes for Confused Old People: A Study of Separation in Social Policy* (London: Longman Group 1972).

Means, Robin. "The Development of Social Services for Elderly People: A Historical Perspective," in *Ageing and Social Policy*, ed. C. Phillips and Allan Walker (London: Gower Aldershot 1986): 87–106.

Medjuck, Sheva, Mary O'Brien, and Carol Tozer. "From Private Responsibility to Public Policy: Women and the Cost of Caregiving to Elderly Kin," *Atlantis* vol. 17, no. 2 (spring-summer 1992): 45–58.

Metress, Seamus. "The History of Irish-American Care of the Aged," *Social Services Review*, vol. 59, no. 1 (March 1985): 18–31.

Minkler, Meredith. "Blaming the Aged Victims: The Politics of Scapegoating in Times of Fixed Conservation," *International Journal of Health Services*, vol. 13 (1983): 155–68.

Mitchinson, Wendy. "Gender and Insanity and Characteristics of the Insane: A Nineteenth-Century Case," *Bulletin Canadienne d'histoire de Medicine / Canadian Bulletin of Medical History*, vol. 4, no. 2 (winter 1987): 97–117.

– "Reasons for Committal to a Mid-Nineteenth-Century Ontario Insane Asylum: The Case of Toronto," in *Essays in the History of Canadian Medicine*, ed. W. Mitchinson and J. McGinnis (Toronto: University of Toronto Press 1988).

Mohl, Raymond. "Poverty in Early America, A Reappraisal: The Case of Eighteenth Century New York City," *New York History*, vol. 50 (1969): 5–27.

– "Three Centuries of American Public Welfare, 1600–1932," *Current History*, vol. 65 (1973): 6–10.

– "The Abolition of Public Outdoor Relief, 1870–1900: A Critique of the Piven and Cloward Thesis," in *Social Welfare or Social Control: Some Historical Reflections on Regulating the Poor*, ed. Walter Trattner (Knoxville: University of Tennessee Press 1983): 35–50.

Montigny, Edgar-André. "Historiography of Destitution: Canadian Historians and Old Age" (paper presented to the Canadian Historical Association Annual Meeting, St Catharines, June 1996).

Moscovitch, Allan and Glenn Drover. "Social Expenditures and the Welfare State: The Canadian Experience in Historical Perspective," in *The Benevolent State: The Growth of Welfare in Canada*, ed. Allan Moscovitch and J. Albert (Toronto: Garamond 1987): 13–43.

Murray, David. "The Cold Hand of Charity: The Court of Quarter Sessions and Poor Relief in the Niagara District, 1828–1841," *Canadian Law in History Conference Papers* (Carleton University 1987): 201–38.

Myles, John. "The Aged, The State and the Structure of Inequality," in *Structured Inequality in Canada*, ed. John Harp and John Hofley (Scarborough, Ont.: Prentice Hall 1980): 317–42.

– *Old Age in the Welfare State: The Political Economy of Public Pensions* (Boston, Mass.: Little, Brown 1984).

– "Social Security and Support of the Elderly: The Western Experience," *Journal of Aging Studies*, vol. 2, no. 4 (winter 1988): 321–37.

Nash, Gary. "Poverty and Poor Relief in Pre-Revolutionary Philadelphia," *William and Mary Quarterly*, vol. 33 (January 1976): 3–30.

Neugarten, Bernice and Dail Neugarten. "Changing Meanings of Age in the Aging Society," in *Our Aging Society: Paradox and Promise*, ed. Alan Pifer and Lydia Bronte (New York: Norton 1986): 33–51.

Newman-Brown, W. "The Receipt of Poor Relief and Family Situation in Aldenham, Hertfordshire, 1630–1690," in *Land, Kinship and Life-Cycle*, ed. Richard Smith (Cambridge, U.K.: Cambridge University Press 1984).

Neysmith, Sheila and Lillian Wells. "Home Care: Who Defines the Priorities," in *An Aging Population: The Challenge for Community Action*, ed. Lillian Wells (Toronto: University of Toronto Press 1991): 96–107.

Noelker, Linda and A. Townsend, "Perceived Caregiving Effectiveness: The Impact of Parental Impairment, Community Resources and Caregiver Characteristics," in *Aging, Health and Family: Long-Term Care*, ed. T. Brubaker (Newbury Park, CA.: Sage Publications 1987).

Northcott, Herbert. *Aging in Alberta: Rhetoric and Reality* (Calgary: Detselig 1992).

O'Brien, Patricia. *Out of Mind, Out of Sight: A History of the Waterford Hospital* (St John's: Waterford Hospital Corp. 1989).

Ontario, Government of. *Redirection of Long-Term Care and Support Services in Ontario: Questions and Answers* (Toronto 1994).

Ontario Nursing Home Association. *The Ontario Nursing Homes Association's Response to the Government's Redirection of Long-Term Care and Support Services in Ontario* (Markham, Ont.: 1992).

Orloff, Ann Shola. *The Politics of Pensions: A Comparative Analysis of Britain, Canada and the United States, 1880–1940* (Madison, Wis.: University of Wisconsin Press 1993).

Pampel, Fred and J.B. Williamson. "Welfare Spending in Advanced Industrial Democracies, 1950–1980," *American Journal of Sociology*, vol. 93 (1988): 1,424–56.

Park, D.C. and J. Wood. "Poor Relief and the County House of Refuge System in Ontario, 1880–1911," *Journal of Historical Geography*, vol. 18, no. 4 (October 1992): 439–55.

Parker. R.A. "An Historical Background to Residential Care," in *Residential Care: The Research Reviewed*, vol. 2 (London: National Institute for Social Work 1988).

Patterson, Norman. "Canadian People: A Criticism," *Canadian Magazine*, vol. 13 (1899).

Pelling, Margaret. "Old Age, Poverty and Disability in Early Modern Norwich: Work, Remarriage and Other Expedients," in *Life, Death and the Elderly: Historical Perspectives*, ed. Margaret Pelling and Richard Smith (London: Routldge 1992): 74–101.

Pelling, Margaret and Richard Smith (eds.). *Life, Death and the Elderly: Historical Perspectives* (London: Routledge 1992): 1–38.

Phillipson, Christopher. "Challenging the "Spectre of Old Age": Community Care for Older People in the 1990's," in *Social Policy Review*, vol. 4, ed. Nickolas Manning and Robert Page (London: Social Policy Association 1992): 111–33.

Pitsula, James. "The Treatment of Tramps in Late-Nineteenth-Century Toronto," Historical Papers (1980): 116–32.

Pollett, P., I. Anderson, and P. O'Connor. "For Better or for Worse: The Experience of Caring for an Elderly Dementing Spouse," *Ageing and Society*, vol. 11 (1991): 443–69.

Pollock, Horatio Milo. *Family Care of Mental Patients* (New York: Arno 1976; reprint of 1936 original).

Quadagno, Jill. *Aging in Early Industrial Society: Work, Family and Social Policy Nineteenth-Century England* (New York: Academic Press 1982).

– "The Transformation of Old Age Security," in *Old Age in a Bureaucratic Society: The Elderly, the Experts and the State in American History*, ed. David Van Tassel and Peter Stearns (New York: Greenwood Press 1986): 129–52.

– "Generational Equality and the Politics of the Welfare State," International Journal of Health Services, vol. 20 (1990): 631–50.

Qureshi, Hazel and Allan Walker. "Caring for Elderly People: The Family and the State," in *Ageing and Social Policy*, ed. C. Phillips and A. Walker (London: Aldershot 1986): 109–27.

Radcliffe, David. "Growing Old in Ontario: A Grey Area," in *New Directions for the Study of Ontario's Past*, ed. David Gagan and Rosemary Gagan (Hamilton Ont.: McMaster University Press 1988): 179–86.

Ramson, Roger and Richard Sutch. "The Labour of Older Americans: Retirement of Men on and off the Job, 1870–1937," *Journal of Economic History*, vol. 46 (1986): 1–30.

– "The Decline of Retirement in the Years Before Social Security: United States Retirement Patterns, 1870–1940," in *Issues in Contemporary Retirement*, ed. R. Campbell and E. Lazear (Stanford, C.A.: Hoover Institution Press 1988): 3–37.

Resnick, Philip. "Neo-Conservatism and Beyond," in *Continuities and Discontinuities: The Political Economy of Social Welfare and Labour Market Policy in Canada*, ed. Andrew Johnson, Stephen McBride and Patrick Smith (Toronto: University of Toronto Press 1994): 25–35.

Reznick, Samuel. "Unemployment, Unrest and Relief in the United States during the Depression of 1893–97," *Journal of Political Economy*, vol. 61 (August 1953): 342–5.

– "Patterns of Thought and Action in an American Depression, 1882–86," *American Historical Review*, vol. 61 (January 1956): 284–306.

Ridler, Niel. "Population Aging: Its Fiscal Impact in Selected OECA Countries." *Canadian Studies in Population*, vol. 11, no. 1 (1984): 47–60.

Rimlinger, Gaston. "Welfare Policy and Economic Development: A Comparative Historical Perspective," *Journal of Economic History*, vol. 26 (December 1966): 556–71.

Robin, Jean. "Family Care of the Elderly in a Nineteenth-Century Devonshire Parish," *Ageing and Society*, vol. 4, no. 4 (1984): 505–16.

Roebuck, Judith. "When Does Old Age Begin? The Evolution of the English Definition," *Journal of Social History*, vol. 12 (1979): 416–28.

Roebuck, Judith and Jane Slaughter. "Ladies and Pensioners: Stereotypes and Public Policy Affecting Old Women in England, 1880–1940," *Journal of Social History*, vol. 13, no. 1 (fall 1979): 105–14.

Rook, Patricia and Schnell, R.L. "Childhood and Charity in Nineteenth-Century British North America," *Histoire Sociale / Social History*, vol. 15 (1982): 157–79.

Rosenberg, Charles. *The Care of Strangers: The Rise of America's Hospital System* (New York: Basic Books 1987).

Rosencrantz, Barbara and Maris Vinovskis. "The Invisible Lunatics: Old Age and Insanity in Mid-Nineteenth-Century Massachusetts," in *Aging and the Elderly: Humanistic Perspectives in Gerontology*, ed. Stuart Spiker, Kathleen Woodward, and David Van Tassel (Atlantic Highlands, N.J.: Humanities Press 1978): 95–125.

Rosenthal, Carolyn. and James Gladstone. "Family Relationships and Support in Later Life." *Journal of Canadian Studies*, vol. 28, no. 1 (spring 1993): 122–38.

Rotella, Elyce and George Alter. "Working Class Debt in Late-Nineteenth-Century United States," *Journal of Family History*, vol. 18, no. 2 (spring 1993): 111–34.

Rothman, David. *The Almshouse Experience: Collected Reports* (New York: Arno Press 1971).

– *Conscience and Convenience: The Asylum and Its Alternatives in Progressive America* (Boston, Mass.: Little, Brown 1980).

Schneider, David. "The Patchwork of Relief in Provincial New York, 1664–1775," *Social Services Review*, vol. 12 (December 1938): 469–94.

Scull, Andrew. *Museums of Madness: The Social Organization of Insanity in Nineteenth-Century England* (London: A. Lane 1979).

– "A Convenient Place to Get Rid of Inconvenient People: The Victorian Lunatic Asylum," in *Buildings and Society*, ed. A.D. King (London: Routledge and Kegan Paul 1980): 37–60.

– "Humanitarianism or Control: Observations on the Historiography of Anglo-American Psychiatry," *Rice University Studies*, vol. 67 (1981): 21–41.

Senior Citizen's Consumer Alliance. *Consumer Report on Long-Term Care Reform* (Toronto 1992).

Serow, William and David Sly. "Trends in the Characteristics of the Oldest Old, 1940–2020," *Journal of Aging Studies*, vol. 2, no. 2 (summer 1988): 145–56.

Shanas, Ethel. "Social Myth as Hypothesis: The Case of the Family Relationships of Old People," *Gerontologist*, vol. 19 (1979): 3–9.

– "Older People and Their Families: The New Pioneers," *Journal of Marriage and the Family*, vol. 42 (1980): 9–15.

Shegog, R.F. *The Impending Crisis of Old Age: A Challenge to Ingenuity* (London: Oxford University Press 1981).

Simmons, Harvey. *From Asylum to Welfare* (Downsview, Ont.: Association for Mental Retardation 1982).

Smith, Daniel Scott. "A Community-Based Sample of the Older Population from the 1800 and 1900 United States Manuscript Census," *Historical Methods*, vol. 11 (1978): 67–74.

– "Old Age and the 'Great Transformation': A New England Case Study," in *Aging and the Elderly: Humanistic Perspectives in Gerontology*, ed. Stuart Spiker, Kathleen Woodward, and David Van Tassel (Atlantic Highlands, N.J.: Humanities Press 1978): 285–302.

– "Life-Course Norms and the Family Systems of Older Americans in 1900," *Journal of Family History*, vol. 4, no. 1 (1979): 285–98.

– "Accounting for Change in the Families of the Elderly in the United States, 1900 to the Present," in *Old Age in a Bureaucratic Society*, ed. David Van Tassel and Peter Stearns (Westport, Conn.: Greenwood Press 1986): 87–109.

Smith, James. "Widowhood and Aging in Traditional English Society," *Ageing and Society*, vol. 4, no. 4 (1984): 429–49.

Smith, Richard. "Kin and Neighbours in a Thirteenth-Century Suffolk Community," *Journal of Family History*, vol. 4, no. 3 (1979): 219–56.

– "The Structured Dependency of the Elderly As a Recent Development: Some Sceptical Historical Thoughts," *Ageing and Society.* vol. 4, no. 4 (1984): 409–28.

– "The Manorial Court and the Elderly Tennant in Late-Medieval England," in *Life, Death and the Elderly: Historical Perspectives*, ed. Margaret Pelling and Richard Smith (London: Routledge 1992): 39–61.

Smith, Stephen. "Death, Dying and the Elderly in Seventeenth-Century England." in *Aging and the Elderly: Humanistic Perspectives in Gerontology*, ed. Stuart Spiker, Kathleen Woodward, and David Van Tassel (Atlantic Highlands, N.J.: Humanities Press 1978): 205–20.

Snell, James. "Filial Responsibility Laws in Canada: A Historical Perspective," *Canadian Journal on Aging*, vol. 9 (1990): 268–77.

– "Maintenance Agreements for the Elderly: Canada, 1900–1951," *Journal*, Canadian Historical Association, (1992): 197–216.

– "The Gendered Construction of Elderly Marriage, 1900–1950," *Canadian Journal on Aging*. vol. 12 (1993): 509–23.

– *Citizen's Wage: The State and the Elderly in Canada, 1900–1951* (Toronto: University of Toronto Press 1996).

Snell, Kieth, and J. Millar. "Lone-Parent Families and the Welfare State: Past and Present," *Continuity and Change*, vol. 2 (1987): 387–422.

Speisman, Stephen. "Munificent Parsons and Municipal Parsimony: Voluntary vs. Public Poor Relief in Nineteenth-Century Toronto," *Ontario History*, vol. 65 (March 1973): 32–49.

Splane, Richard. *Social Welfare in Ontario, 1791–1893: A Study of Public Welfare Administration* (Toronto: University of Toronto Press 1965).

Stannard, David. "Growing Up and Growing Old: Dilemmas of Aging in Bureaucratic America," in *Aging and the Elderly: Humanistic Perspectives in Gerontology*, ed. Stuart Spiker, Kathleen Woodward, and David Van Tassel (Atlantic Highlands, N.J.: Humanities Press 1978): 9–22.

Stearns, Peter. "Old Women: Some Historical Observations," *Journal of Family History*, vol. 5 (1980): 44–57.

Stewart, Gordon. *The Origins of Canadian Politics: A Comparative Approach* (Vancouver: University of British Columbia Press 1986).

Stewart, Stormi. "The Elderly Poor in Rural Ontario: Inmates of the Wellington County House of Industry, 1877–1907," *Journal*, Canadian Historical Association (1992): 217–34.

Stokes, Mary. "Local Government in the Shadow of the Law: The Municipal Corporation as Legal Actor in Canada West/Ontario, 1850–1870," unpublished paper, University of Western Ontario, 1987.

– "Petitions to the Legislative Assembly of Ontario from Local Governments, 1867–1877: A Case Study in Legislative Participation," *Law and History Review*, vol. 11, no. 1 (spring 1993): 145–80.

Stone, Leroy and Michael Maclean. *Future Income Prospects for Canada's Senior Citizen's* (Toronto: Institute for Research on Public Policy 1979).

Strong, Margaret. *Public Welfare Administration in Canada* (Chicago, Ill.: University of Chicago Press 1930).

Struthers, James. "Regulating the Elderly: Old Age Pensions and the Formation of a Pension Bureaucracy in Ontario, 1929–1945," *Journal*, Canadian Historical Association (1992): 235–56.

- "The Provincial Welfare State and Social Policy in Ontario," *Journal of Canadian Studies*, vol. 27, no. 1 (spring 1993): 136–46.
- *The Limits of Affluence: Welfare in Ontario, 1920–70* (Toronto: University of Toronto Press 1994).
- "A Nice Homelike Atmosphere: Aging and Long-Term Care in Post-World War Two Ontario" (paper presented to the Second Carleton Conference on the History of the Family, Ottawa 1994).

Synge, Jane. "Work and Family Support Patterns of the Aged in the Early Twentieth Century," in *Aging in Canada*, ed. Victor Marshall (Don Mills, Ont.: Fitzhenry and Whiteside 1980): 135–44.

Tarman, Vera Ingird. "Institutional Care and Health Policy for the Elderly," in *Sociology of Health Care in Canada*, ed. Bolaria Singh and Harleg Dickenson (Toronto: Harcourt Brace Javonovitch 1988): 244–57.
- *Privatization and Health Care: The Case of Ontario Nursing Homes* (Toronto: Garamond Press 1990).

Thane, Pat. "The History of Provision for the Elderly to 1929," in *Ageing in Modern Society: Contemporary Approaches*, ed. Dorothy Jerome (London: Croom Helm 1983): 191–9.
- "The Growing Burden of an Aging Population," *Journal of Public Policy*, vol. 7, no. 4 (1987): 373–87.
- "The Debate on the Declining Birth-Rate in Britain: The 'Menace' of an Ageing Population, 1920–1950's," *Continuity and Change*, vol. 5 (1990): 283–305.

Thomas, Donna. *The Problem of the Aged Poor: Social Reform in Late-Victorian England* (Edmonton: University of Alberta 1969).

Thomas, Kieth. "Age and Authority in Modern England," *Proceedings of the British Academy*, vol. 62 (1976): 3–16.

Thomson, David. "Age Reporting by the Elderly and the Nineteenth-Century Census," *Local Population Studies*, vol. 25 (1980): 13–25.
- "Workhouse to Nursing Home: Residential Care of Elderly People in England Since 1848," *Ageing and Society*, vol. 3, no. 1 (March 1983): 43–70.
- "The Decline of Social Welfare: Falling State Support for the Iderly since Early Victorian Times," *Ageing and Society*, vol. 4, no. 4 (1984): 451–82.
- " 'I Am Not My Father's Keeper': Families and the Elderly in Nineteenth-Century England," *Law and History Review*, vol. 2, no. 2 (fall 1984): 265–86.
- "Welfare and Historians," in *The World We Have Gained*, ed. L. Bonfield, R. Smith, and K. Wrightson (New York: Basil Blackwell 1986): 355–78.
- "The Elderly in an Urban-Industrial Society: England 1750 to the Present," in *An Aging World: Dilemma and Challenges for Law and Social Policy*, ed. John Eekelaar and David Pearl (London: Claredon Press 1989): 55–61.
- "The Welfare of the Elderly in the Past: A Family or Community Responsibility," in *Life, Death and the Elderly: Historical Perspectives*, ed. Margaret Pelling and Richard Smith (London: Routledge 1991): 194–221.

– *Selfish Generations? How Welfare States Grow Old* (Wellington, New Zealand: Whitehorse Press 1996).

Tibbles, Lance. "Medical and Legal Aspects of Competency As Affected by Old Age," in *Aging and the Elderly: Humanistic Perspectives in Gerontology*, ed. Stuart Spiker, Kathleen Woodward, and David Van Tassel (Atlantic Highlands, N.J.: Humanities Press 1978): 127–52.

Tolany, Stewart and Avery Guest. "Childlessness in a Transitional Population: The United States at the Turn of the Century," *Journal of Family History*, vol. 7 (1982): 200–19.

Townsend, Peter. "The Structured Dependency of the Elderly: A Creation of Social Policy in the Twentieth-Century," *Ageing and Society*, vol. 1 (1981): 5–28.

– "Ageism and Social Policy," in *Ageing and Social Policy: A Critical Assessment*, ed. Allan Walker and C. Phillips (London: Gower Aldershot 1986): 15–44.

Troyansky, David. *Old Age in the Old Regime: Image and Experience in Eighteenth-Century France* (London: Cornell Press 1989).

– "The Older Person in the Western World: From the Middle Ages to the Industrial Revolution," in *Handbook of the Humanities and Aging*, ed. Thomas Cole, David Van Tassel, and Robert Kastenbaum (New York: Springer Publications 1992): 40–61.

Tuke, David Hack. *The Insane in the United States and Canada* (New York: Arno Press 1973; reprint of 1885 original).

Ulrich, Laurel Thatcher. *Good Wives: Image and Reality in the Lives of Women in New England, 1650–1750* (New York: Alfred Knopf 1982).

– *A Midwife's Tale: The Life of Martha Ballard, Based on Her Diary, 1785–1812* (New York: Vintage Books 1991).

Vallin, Jacques, "Mortality in Europe from 1720 to 1914: Long-Term Trends and Changes in Patterns by Age and Sex," in *The Decline of Mortality in Europe*, ed. R. Schofield, R. Reher, and A. Bideau (Oxford: Claraden Press 1991): 38–67.

Valverde, Marianna. *The Age of Light, Soap and Water: Moral Reform in English Canada, 1885–1925* (Toronto: McClelland and Stewart 1991).

Von Kondratowitz, Hans Joachim. "The Medicalization of Old Age: Continuity and Change in Germany from the Late-Eighteenth to the Early Twentieth-Century," in *Life, Death and The Elderly: Historical Perspectives*, ed. Margaret Pelling and Richard Smith (London: Routledge 1991): 134–64.

Wales, Thomas. "Poverty, Poor Relief and the Life-Cycle: Some Evidence from Seventeenth-Century Norfolk," in *Land, Kinship and Life Cycle*, ed. Richard Smith (Cambridge, U.K.: Cambridge University Press 1984).

Walker, Allan. "The Social Creation of Poverty and Dependency in Old Age," *Journal of Social Policy*, vol. 9 (1980): 45–75.

– "Towards a Political Economy of Old Age," *Ageing and Society*, vol. 1, no. 1 (March 1981): 73–94.

– "Pensions and the Production of Poverty in Old Age, 1970's–1980's," in *Ageing and Social Policy: A Critical Assessment*, ed. Allan Walker and C. Phillips (London: Grover Aldershot 1986).

– "The Relationship Between the Family and the State in the Care of Older People," *Canadian Journal on Aging*, vol. 10, no. 2 (1991): 94–112.

– "Thatcherism and the New Politics of Old Age," in *State, Labour Markets and the Future of Old Age Policy*, ed. John Myles and Jill Quadagno (Philadelphia, PA.: Temple University Press 1991): 19–35.

– "The Future of Long-Term Care in Canada: A British Perspective," *Canadian Journal on Aging*, vol. 14 (1995): 437–46.

Wall, Richard. "The Residential Segregation of the Elderly: A Comparison over Time," *Ageing and Society*, vol. 4 (1984): 483–503.

– "Leaving Home and Living Alone: An Historical Perspective," *Population Studies*, vol. 43 (1989): 369–89.

– "Relationships Between Generations in British Families: Past and Present," in *Families and Households: Divisions and Change*, ed. C. Marsh and S. Arber (London: Macmillan 1992): 63–86.

Wallace, Elizabeth. "Old Age Security in Canada," *Canadian Journal of Economics and Political Science*, vol. 18 (1952): 125–34.

Walton, John. "Lunacy and the Industrial Revolution: A Study of Asylum Admissions in Lancashire, 1848–49," *Journal of Social History*, vol 13 (1979–80): 1–22.

– "The Treatment of Pauper Lunatics in Victorian England: The Case of Lancaster Asylum, 1816–70," in *Madhouses, Mad Doctors and Madmen: The Social History of Psychiatry in the Victorian Era*, ed. Andrew Scull (Philadelphia, PA.: University of Pennsylvania Press 1981): 166–201.

– "Casting Out and Bringing Back in Victorian England: Pauper Lunatics, 1840–1870," in *The Anatomy of Madness, vol 2: Essays in the History of Psychiatry*, ed. W.F. Bynum, R. Porter, and M. Shepherd (London: Tavistock Publications 1985): 132–47.

Warnes, Anthony. "Being Old, Old People and the Burdens of Burden," *Ageing and Society*, vol. 13, no. 3 (September 1993): 297–338.

Warsh, Cheryl Krasnick. *Moments of Unreason: The Practice of Canadian Psychiatry and the Homewood Retreat, 1883–1923* (Montreal: McGill-Queen's University Press 1987).

Watt, Susan. "Models of Family in Health Policy for the Aged," *Canadian Review of Social Policy*, vol. 25 (1990): 33–46.

Weiler, Sue. "Family Security or Social Security: The Family and the Elderly in New York State During the 1920's," *Journal of Family History*, vol. 11, no. 1 (spring 1986): 77–95.

– "Industrial Scrap-heap: Employment Patterns and Change for the Aged in the 1920's," *Social Science History*, vol. 13, no. 1 (spring 1989): 65–88.

Williams, Idris. *Caring for Elderly People in the Community* (London: Chapman and Hall 1986).

Williamson, John B. "Old Age Relief Policies Prior to 1900: The Trend Towards Restrictiveness," *American Journal of Economics and Sociology*, vol. 43, no. 3 (1984): 369–84.

Willianson, John B., Judith Shindul, and Linda Evans. *Aging and Public Policy: Social Control or Social Justice?* (Springfield, Ill.: Charles Thomas 1985).

Williamson, John B., L. Evans, and L. Powell. *The Politics of Aging: Power and Policy* (Springfield, Ill.: Charles Thomas 1982).

Wright, S.J. "The Elderly and the Bereaved in Eighteenth-Century Ludlow," in *Life, Death and the Elderly: Historical Perspectives*, ed. Margaret Pelling and Richard Smith (London: Routledge 1991): 102–34.

Zainaldin, J.S. and P. Tyor. "Asylums and Society: An Approach to Industrial Change," *Journal of Social History*, vol. 13 (1979–80): 23–48.

Zaretsky, Eli. "The Place of the Family in the Origins of the Welfare State," in *Rethinking the Family: Some Feminist Questions*, ed. B. Thorne (New York: Longman 1982): 188–224.

Index